Dental Reception and
Supervisory Management

Dental Reception and Supervisory Management

Second Edition

Glenys Bridges MCIPD, FBDPMA, RDN, dip. DPM
Managing Partner of Glenys Bridges
and Partners Training and Development

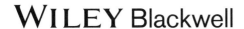

Registered Office
John Wiley & Sons, Inc., 111 River Street, Hoboken, NJ 07030, USA
John Wiley & Sons Ltd, The Atrium, Southern Gate, Chichester, West Sussex, PO19 8SQ, UK

Editorial Office
9600 Garsington Road, Oxford, OX4 2DQ, UK

For details of our global editorial offices, customer services, and more information about Wiley products visit us at www.wiley.com.

Wiley also publishes its books in a variety of electronic formats and by print-on-demand. Some content that appears in standard print versions of this book may not be available in other formats.

Library of Congress Cataloging-in-Publication Data

Names: Bridges, Glenys, 1956– author.
Title: Dental reception and supervisory management / Glenys Bridges.
Description: Second edition. | Hoboken, NJ : Wiley-Blackwell, [2019] | Includes bibliographical references and index. |
Identifiers: LCCN 2018051417 (print) | LCCN 2018052026 (ebook) | ISBN 9781119513063 (Adobe PDF) | ISBN 9781119513025 (ePub) | ISBN 9781119513087 (pbk.)
Subjects: | MESH: Dental Auxiliaries | Practice Management, Dental–organization & administration
Classification: LCC RK58 (ebook) | LCC RK58 (print) | NLM WU 90 | DDC 617.6/0068–dc23
LC record available at https://lccn.loc.gov/2018051417

Cover Design: Wiley
Cover Image: © Matthias Tunger / Getty Images

Set in 10/12pt Warnock by SPi Global, Pondicherry, India
Printed in Singapore by C.O.S. Printers Pte Ltd

10 9 8 7 6 5 4 3 2 1

Contents

Preface

This book focuses on the range of knowledge and skills that receptionists and supervisory managers need to offer friendly, patient-focused front of house and administration services, which support and enhance the reputation of the practice and the work of their clinical colleagues as well as providing patients with oral health gains.

This book aims to detail the impact upon dental administration of the ongoing development of regulations intended to ensure that standards of dental care are continuously improving. This ongoing development culture has resulted in considerable changes in dental team roles and involves the likes of extended duties for dental care professionals and laws to regulate data security and protection.

The reception role was always a challenging one, calling for a range of learned and innate skills as covered in Chapter 2 of this book. Alongside the receptionists' formally learned skills, their innate skills are a reflection of their personality and serve to create the personality that the practice projects every day to all who come across it.

In Chapter 3, the focus is on the front-of-house marketing role, looking at how information about the local market can be collected and considering numerous ways that receptionists can use that information to raise the profile of the practice within the local community.

Financial aspects of reception, aspects of consent linked to the financial aspects of treatment, are the subject matter for Chapter 4. Financial misunderstandings are frequently the cause of complaints and patient dissatisfaction. Receptionists have an important role to play in ensuring there is clarity and transparency in financial matters relating to the dental services offered to patients.

Staff selection is the focus of Chapter 5. How to select the right people during recruitment activity as well as the main factors to consider when allocating work and selecting team members for specific responsibilities are discussed.

In Chapter 6, quality management is explored – the ideology that has led to the care quality standards each practice must meet. The chapter then looks at practical ways these management approaches can be applied to enhance the quality of care for patients and the ability of dental workplaces to cultivate job satisfaction and team retention.

Enabling a group of people to come together and become a collaborative team calls for a range of communication skills as covered in Chapter 7, in which considerations of aspects of IQ and emotional intelligence (EQ) are explored along with techniques for responding to challenging behaviour and workplace bullying.

Chapter 8 extends the communication theme and looks at how the reception lead can structure methods of information sharing, the role of meetings to analyse significant events and learn from experience using reflective practice.

Safety and well-being is the focus for Chapter 9. Here we look at important safeguarding requirements to ensure that should a member of the reception team have concerns for a child or vulnerable adult, they are aware of what the practice expects them to do and are able to act swiftly in a preventive or safeguarding role.

The patient journey is a term that is well established in dental speak and is the subject of Chapter 10. It covers a wide range of aspects of the patient experience and looks at ways the practice can give their patients something extra that shows they value their patients and understand their needs and concerns. This topic is extended in Chapter 11 to look at the newest team role – that of care coordinator. There are many ways that practices apply this role. In most cases, the role is closely linked to the reception team, so they can access clinical expertise to answer patients' questions and ensure that patients can give informed consent to every aspect of their care and treatment.

Chapter 12 looks at aspects of computer technology and the need for every team member to be aware of the required security measures for the prevention of cyberattacks.

About the Companion Website

Don't forget to visit the companion website for this book:

www.wiley.com/go/bridges/dental

There you will find valuable material designed to enhance your learning, including:

- Activities
- PowerPoint presentation

Scan this QR code to visit the companion website.

1

The Developing World of Dental Care Services

History of the Nonclinical Dental Team

Teamwork is an essential part of modern dentistry and is critical to the provision of high-quality, patient-focused dental care. It is no longer an option for dental practitioners to manage the clinical and regulatory issues of their business without the support of a team. This has led to the introduction of more defined leadership and management roles and the need for a whole-team approach to develop and maintain dental services that are compliant with legal and ethical requirements. It has also led to legislation and regulations to govern the care and business aspects of dentistry.

Modern dental care has evolved from innovations and regulations that have their roots in the Medical Act of 1858. Before gaining recognition as a profession, dentistry was a branch of the medical profession, but under the terms of the Medical Act, Queen Victoria granted a charter to the Royal College of Surgeons to award licences in dentistry. Two years later, 43 candidates passed the first examination to receive the Licentiate of Dental Surgery.

In 1878, the first Dentists Act required a register of dentists to be kept by the General Medical Council. Previously, there had been no requirement for those carrying out acts of dentistry to hold recognized qualifications. Despite the Dentist Act, barber-surgeons and blacksmiths continued to extract teeth in public places with little regard for hygiene or patient care. This changed with the enactment of the Dentist Act 1921. To protect the public, the Act defined 'acts of dentistry' and limited acts of dentistry to individuals with a recognised qualification and who are registered with the government-appointed professional lead body.

The next significant milestone for the dental profession was the introduction of the National Health Service (NHS) in 1948. Most dentists worked alone, often from part of their own home converted into a dental surgery. The range of treatments delivered by general dental practitioners (GDPs) was limited, with complex procedures being referred to a dental hospital. At this time, most dentists preferred to mix their materials. Since air turbines were yet to be invented, a simple saliva ejector was sufficient to keep the treatment area dry. The only assistance dentists required was in the form of someone to answer the doorbell, book appointments with patients (very few people had a telephone, so the phone was not a consideration), and complete the National Health Service (NHS) paperwork. In many cases, the dentist's wife or the daughter of a well-off

Dental Reception and Supervisory Management, Second Edition. Glenys Bridges.
© 2019 John Wiley & Sons Ltd. Published 2019 by John Wiley & Sons Ltd.
Companion website: www.wiley.com/go/bridges/dental

family (who were hoping that their daughter would find a professional husband through her work) fulfilled these duties. In this way, the earliest receptionist role was created.

In the 1950s, a new generation of dental equipment was being developed, such as the high-speed drills that became standard equipment by the 1960s. Belt-driven drills were replaced by air-driven, water-cooled, high-speed drills. Because of the water coolants that accompanied this equipment, it was necessary for someone to work alongside the dentist to remove excess water for the patient's comfort and to keep the operating area dry. By the late 1950s, in some avant-garde, high-tech practices, the four-handed style of dentistry was growing in popularity.

By the late 1960s, dentistry was experiencing a period of rapid change. As a result, the role of support staff began to change. A new trend emerged for dentists to work in multi-practitioner practices. At the same time, more and more patients were contacting dental practices by telephone. This meant that one-person assisting was no longer adequate. There was a need for someone to work chairside while someone else answered the phone, managed the appointment book, and collected patients' payments. Under these conditions, the multiskilled nurse-receptionist role came into its own in the delivery of patient care.

Another wave of change began in the early 1990s, leading to the development of nonclinical skills. This was driven primarily by two factors: computerisation and patient demands. Computer skills were needed to enable dental businesses to achieve the best value from their considerable investment in equipment, and meanwhile, nonclinical client care skills were essential as the service aspect of the National Health Service came to the fore. The surgery role also became more involved, with an increased range of skills, knowledge, and qualifications being required to provide higher-quality dental care.

A further impact of the changes of the 1990s was the development of another team role: the practice manager. The number of practice managers in the post has grown rapidly since 1992 and continues to grow. The impetus for this is the massive and far-reaching changes in the delivery of primary dental care services, including initiatives such as clinical governance and continuous changes in general and employment law. Today, management decisions previously taken by governing authorities on as fee scales and the availability of services are managed in-house, sometimes with little or no guidance. This creates a substantial amount of extra work. Clinically trained practitioners find that running a small business places enormous demands on their time and resources. As management tasks are not revenue generating, they represent a drain on practice resources. Therefore, a manager is essential for overseeing the tactical management of the practice. To fulfil this role, practice managers need a good knowledge of how the practice works as well as the needs of both the team and patients.

The new millennium has seen a significant increase in legislation and regulation for dental teams. In 2013 the General Dental Council revised the Standards for the Dental Team.[1] This includes the following nine principles, along with guidance for their implementation:

1) Put patients' interests first.
2) Communicate effectively with patients.

---

[1] General Dental Council (2013). *Standards for the Dental Team.* https://standards.gdc-uk.org/Assets/pdf/Standards%20for%20the%20Dental%20Team.pdf

3) Obtain valid consent.
4) Maintain and protect patients' information.
5) Have a clear and effective complaints procedure.
6) Work with colleagues in a way that is in patients' best interests.
7) Maintain, develop, and work with your professional knowledge and skills.
8) Raise concerns if patients are at risk.
9) Make sure your behaviour maintains patients' confidence in you and the dental profession.

These standards set out ethical requirements. Many of these requirements impact the standards of the work of nonclinical aspects of patients care, so the practice must develop roles and procedures based on the standards to ensure that those who are not General Dental Council (GDC) registrants are also obliged to meet statutory, regulatory requirements.

In 2008, the Health and Social Care Act introduced far-reaching legislation aimed at setting fundamental standards for the delivery of health care that is:

- Safe
- Effective
- Caring
- Responsive
- Well led

This legislation applies to all providers of health and social care. Providers are required to register with the authoritative body with jurisdiction in their region, and to name a registered provider and a registered manager who will be responsible for maintaining the required care standards. Inspectors with the power to act to protect patients' interests will visit providers' premises to ensure that the required standards are consistently being met by each member of the team.

Since the millennium, the practice manager role has developed considerably, in response to developments in the structure of the dental profession. Substantial changes in regulation have affected business aspects of dentistry. The role of practice managers will continue to develop due to the range of financial demands associated with corporate dentistry, government policy on care quality standards, and the increased professional status for dental care professionals (DCPs). Today, increasing numbers of practice managers are practice owners or are shareholders in their practice.

Today's DCPs are highly skilled and, increasingly, are highly qualified dental professionals. However, the skills and aptitude required to be a good nurse are not wholly the same as those needed to be an equally good receptionist. The nurse-receptionist role is evolving into two different and highly skilled DCP roles. With the introduction of mandatory dental nurse qualifications, practices question the deployment of qualified nurses at the reception desk, carrying out work for which their qualifications are not required.

Patients are becoming increasingly vocal about their care and treatment. The General Dental Council sets standards for informed consent. Patients are asking questions more often, and dental professionals have a duty to provide accurate responses in a format that patients can understand sufficiently well to make informed choices. The practice manager can ensure that responses are initiated by clinicians and standardized amongst the team.

We can expect that the practice manager's role will continue to change as developments occur within the profession. On reflection, we can see that dental health care has changed dramatically over the last century and is continuing to evolve. As a result, yet another role is emerging, that of the care coordinator. This role will enable dentists to offer a full range of patient education services, with the knowledge that their patients can make informed choices of the treatment options available to them. The care coordinator role will be an important step in the continuing development of dental care.

The Ethos and Ethics of Dental Care

Ethos

In the earliest recorded accounts, dentistry is described as a healing art. Advances throughout the twentieth century changed the profession dramatically and created today's culture of dental care, and today modern dentistry is an exact, high-tech science. Before becoming a self-regulated profession, dentistry had its share of amusing folk remedies, colourful quacks, and cults. Now dentists must observe the highest ethical standards by placing patients' interests first and acting to protect them.

Historically, most health-care professions have focused on curative care. Dentistry was one of the first health-care professions to focus on prevention and patient education, aiming to create awareness of the causes of dental problems and to enable patients to make lifestyle changes to prevent dental disease. Today, most general medical practitioners now offer their patients regular health assessments and lifestyle checks, taking an approach tried and tested within the dental profession for decades.

The ethos of modern dentistry developed throughout the last century, guided by successive versions of the Dentists Act. The Dentists Act of 1921 was a milestone in the profession's development. This Act ended an apprenticeship system where both qualified and unqualified dentists and medical practitioners shared the practice of dentistry. William Guy, who introduced this Act, led the drive to stop dental care being delivered by unqualified dentists. He was conscious of the need to protect the public from the dangers of dental treatments performed by unqualified practitioners and devoted his energies to arousing his colleagues from their lethargy and persuading them that legislation prohibiting unqualified practice was essential for the protection of the public.

The 1921 Dentists Act made sure that only registered and qualified dentists were permitted to practice. Since then, a whole range of laws, standards, and regulations has been introduced to shape the profession. Other milestones in the development of the dental profession were the introduction of the National Health Service in 1948, and the establishment of the General Dental Council in 1956.

Ethics

The GDC's role is to protect patients and regulate the dental team. The GDC protects patients by promoting confidence in dental professionals through the enforcement of ethical standards of practice and conduct. Adherence to a formally agreed set of values is a fundamental aspect of professionalism. The concept of ethical codes specifying standards of behaviour can be tracked back as far as Moses and the 10 Commandments.

Early Grecian civilisation is recognized as the birthplace of Western ethics. Socrates challenged the right of the strong to oppress the weak and taught that the strong should uphold the rights of the weak. This was not readily accepted in early Greek society, and in around 400 BC Socrates was put to death for 'corrupting the youth of Athens'. Socrates angered the authorities of the day by urging individuals to make reasoned distinctions between what is morally right and what is in their own best interests.

The French philosopher Descartes is the father of modern Western ethics. In his book *Le Monde*, published in 1633, he aimed to 'encourage all who had the good sense to think for themselves', and he offered guiding principles and a moral code on which to base thinking, as follows.

Guiding Principles

1) Accept nothing as true that is not self-evident.
2) Divide problems into their simplest parts.
3) Solve problems by proceeding from the simple to the complex.
4) Check and recheck the reasoning.

Moral Code

1) Obey local customs and laws.
2) Make decisions based on the best evidence.
3) Change desires, rather than trying to change the world.
4) Always seek the truth.

Although lifestyles and moral standards have changed considerably since 1633, these guiding principles still provide a basis for building trust and respect.

The GDC publishes ethical guidance for the dental profession and sets guiding principles in the following six fundamental principles of ethical practice:

1) Put patients' interests first and act to protect them. This principle sets out the responsibility of GDC registrants to work within the scope of their knowledge and keep accurate patient records.
2) Respect patients' dignity and choices. Here, the requirement to treat patients with equality and dignity and give them all the information required to make decisions is outlined.
3) Protect patients' confidential information. This sets the standards for use and disclosure of information held about patients and outlines the circumstances under which such information can be disclosed.
4) Cooperate with other members of the dental team and other health-care colleagues in the interests of patients. Protocols for communications between health-care professionals for the best interests of patients are defined.
5) Maintain professional knowledge and competence. Dental professionals should keep their knowledge, skills, and professional performance under continuous review and identify their limitations as well as their strengths.
6) Be trustworthy. Dental professionals should act fairly and honestly in all their professional and personal dealings.

Maintaining acceptable standards of behaviour for each of these principles requires all members of the dental team to be fully aware of their roles and responsibilities. Guidance is in place to provide clear and detailed definitions, and direct the dental team to work most effectively.

You can find the most up-to-date information on the GDC website, http://www.gdc-uk.org.

Dental Reception Skills

It is widely accepted that the receptionist is the crucial link between the public and the practice team. High-quality, consistent administrative services are, without exception, the result of clearly defined systems, backed up by training and resources for those operating those systems.

Methodical working systems portray an image of professionalism. Receptionists usually work under pressure, needing to multitask in a hectic environment. Therefore, agreed, structured working patterns are vital to avoid chaos. With experience, receptionists can learn to follow systems designed for working effectively under pressure.

Good receptionists learn to judge and respond to the moods of patients, dentists, and work colleagues. When practical and interpersonal skills are blended, the result is confident, competent receptionist services. The role of the reception supervisor is to apply practical skills in ways that support the development of those skills in the people whose work they supervise.

The familiar role of the nurse/receptionist is long established in the dental sector. However, all too often, ongoing training focuses on clinical rather than administration skills. Those skills are frequently sidelined and undervalued, but patients' perceptions of the quality of their dental care are more often based on customer care rather than clinical care standards. The will to ensure that every patient's journey is smooth and seamless must be embedded in every dental practice.

In every business sector, the success of small businesses is dependent on good operating systems. Computerisation enables businesses to operate standard systems much more easily than before. Modern computer systems allow operators to access data to analyse performance and relative costs. Many practices use computerised appointment books and, as a result, can analyse attendance and failure rates. They can produce accurate information about patient numbers and treatment uptake. Without this type of information, practice administration cannot accurately identify trends and plan timely responses.

It is not only patients who become stressed: colleagues too can feel under pressure, so taking time to consider how other people are feeling can go a long way in reducing workplace stress. When the appointment book runs late, stress comes to the forefront. Here the receptionist should be aware of the need to liaise effectively between the surgery and the patient, keeping everyone informed and maintaining goodwill. A good receptionist learns to judge the mood of patients, dentists, and work colleagues.

When speaking to patients over the telephone, the receptionist should sound friendly and efficient and maintain a positive tone. Your practice should set telephone protocols to reflect the ideals of the practice, which are observed by all members of the team when answering the telephone.

An important aspect of the practice is the atmosphere surrounding the reception area. Reception working areas should be kept uncluttered and tidy always, as this shows competence and control of your work environment. This calls for methodical working systems, which are vital to add professionalism to administrative services. Learning to work under pressure comes with experience.

Role of the Receptionist

The role of the receptionist will vary from practice to practice. The team role of the receptionist is outlined by the British Dental Receptionists Association in broad terms:

> As part of the practice team, to assist in the provision of dental care services.... To embrace the organisation, implementation and delivery of dental services by developing patient care procedures to ensure maximum contribution to the practice's profitability, in line with GDC guidelines and practice policies.

This is carried out through the following tasks:

- Open and close the practice each working day.
- Welcome patients and visitors and direct them to appropriate waiting areas.
- Notify providers (dentist or hygienist) of each patient's arrival.
- Review adherence to schedule and remind the provider and inform patients of excessive delays.
- Anticipate patients' anxieties.
- Answer patients' questions.
- Arrange appointments in person or by telephone.
- Enter and retrieve patient records.
- Send out recalls.
- Receive and redirect all incoming telephone calls as appropriate.
- Operate the central paging and music system.
- Operate the computer system in observation of legal and ethical guidelines.
- Monitor the hazard warning systems and notify the appropriate person of occurrences.
- Sell sundry products at patients' requests.
- Calculate and collect patient charges.
- Note feedback from patients.
- Complete NHS claims.
- Respond to emergencies in line with practice policy.
- Participate in professional development activities.
- Attend regular staff meetings.

Perform these and other related duties necessary to maintain a high standard of patient care with due regard for patient confidentiality.

Personal Skillsets

The receptionist's job description should be agreed and written down and should be reviewed as part of the appraisal process. Any areas in which improvements are required can be addressed, and an action plan agreed to strengthen areas of underperformance.

The receptionist plays an extremely important role in ensuring the smooth running of the practice. Because it is vital that work is carried out to the highest possible standard, employers are advised to look for the following skills when recruiting reception staff.

To begin with, the receptionist must be organized and efficient. This will result in work being carried out in an effective and efficient manner. Employers know the effects of a badly run reception; it will have repercussions throughout the practice. An organized reception also looks more professional to patients and may make nervous patients feel at ease, whereas a chaotic workplace appears unprofessional and may increase their anxiety.

Good timekeeping is also essential. The receptionist needs to be on the premises in good time to greet the first patients of the session.

Receptionists should be observant. It is important to monitor the comings and goings of patients and to keep an eye on the waiting room. If a patient has been waiting for a long time, an apology must be made, and the situation should be brought to the attention of the dentist.

Excellent communication skills are essential. If communication is lacking between team members, it often means things get forgotten, missed, or not done properly. It is equally important for the dental receptionist to be able to communicate with the patients. At times this will involve using a sympathetic, caring manner, whereas at other times assertiveness will be required. Nervous patients need a reassuring tone of voice to help calm their nerves, but difficult issues or complaints may need to be dealt with using a more assertive approach. Speaking in a clear voice is very important so that people can fully understand what you are saying. Listening can be just as important as speaking, and if a message needs passing on, its meaning must be retained so it makes sense to the person for whom it is intended.

Excellent administrative skills are needed to ensure that all reception duties are prioritized and completed with competence. At times the receptionist will be required to make decisions within the framework of the practice rules and should be confident enough to do so.

Being computer literate is also an advantage, as most dental practices now rely on computer systems for booking appointments and typing referral letters.

Customer care skills are vital, especially a friendly disposition which must be retained even at the busiest of times and when working under pressure.

To ensure patients' dental experiences are positive, receptionists must have the following skills and abilities:

Communication	Being comfortable with communicating with all types of people.
Empathy	Being able to see matters from the patient's point of view.
Organization	Ability to deliver streamlined and friendly services.
Language	Ability to speak clearly and use appropriate language.

With these abilities in place, receptionists project the image of being confident and competent dental professionals who take pride in their work.

Supervisory Management Skills

In today's dental practices, everyone needs to be committed to the concept of *whole team professionalism*. This means each member of the dental team needs to have a working knowledge of the principles of professionalism, leading to adherence to a set of values comprising both a formally agreed-on code of conduct and the informal expectations of colleagues and society. The key obligations are to act in the patients' best interests, giving full respect to society's health needs. When each person in the team is fully committed to these standards, the role of practice manager is straightforward.

In many cases, managers are finding workers increasingly difficult to manage, especially those who do not respect rank or rules and are more concerned about themselves, their families, and the deals they can make for their own benefit than with loyalty or commitment to standards of professionalism. At times managers feel they are in a stressful tug-of-war. On one side are the demands of professionalism, and on the other side the demands of employees. In this environment, it can feel like they are continuously trying to define their level of authority. The title of *practice manager* does not guarantee respect, just as drawing up policy does not ensure implementation, and delegation of work does not ensure the desired results.

Never have the skills of management been so frequently studied and defined as over recent years, resulting in the strongly contested debate over the merits of hands-on versus hands-off management approaches. The hands-on approach can be useful in maintaining strong work standards, but it can also be used as a cloaking device for the manager's shortfalls in being able to train and motivate workers to be self-starters. By contrast, managers who use a hands-off approach should be alert to the fact that the result may be a severe case of undermanagement with resulting deterioration in worker–employer relationships and a lowering of work standards. When asked, managers who preferred this approach claim they are 'empowering' their people by remaining hands off. Nobody wants to be micromanaged; the feeling that the boss is breathing down your neck is claustrophobic. However, undermanagement results when managers fail to keep informed about the details of their team members' tasks and responsibilities, and they neglect to provide clear direction and support or to hold individuals accountable for their performance. Failure to provide these management basics leads to a downward spiral, which is devastating to both the credibility of managers and the motivation of employees.

HOT Management (Bruce Tulgan)

One approach aims to avoid the pitfalls of both hands-on and hands-off management. The term *HOT management* is used to describe a hands-on transactional management style, which requires managers to be:

Informed	Fully aware of both the legal and ethical obligations placed on dental professionals and understanding their teams' challenges and triumphs.
Comfortable	With their role and justly confident in their management competence, and with adequate support mechanisms for managers and the teams they manage.
Understanding	Having empathy for the needs of both patients and employees, leading to the recognition of people's problems and achievements.
Relaxed	In their approach to personnel management, using a calm 'can-do' approach supported by policies and protocols to provide an equitable working environment.
Confident	Showing confidence when dealing with difficult people and circumstances.
Leaders	Effective leaders give clear direction and set standards by example while supporting all the team to meet those standards.
In touch	With team members and aware of each person's value to the team.
Sociable	Networking with colleagues in the dental community, sharing ideas and experiences, and considering them as allies, not competitors.
Innovative	Not stuck in a rut; prepared to make carefully thought-out changes.
Successful	Business success brings rewards on all levels; 'work smarter', making the best use of the team's skills and enjoying the rewards.

The nature of management lies between a science and an art. This requires managers to have a good aptitude for the objective scientific skills such as managing income and expenditure, organizing practicalities, and setting the policies, procedures, and protocols to create equitable, consistent, and robust workplace environments. Also, they need a range of soft management skills such as providing pastoral care to build loyalty, motivation, and a sense of belonging into the team. On their own, excellence in only one of these types of skills leads to poor team performance: good management is a balance of both aptitudes.

Specific Duties of a Supervisor

The specific duties of reception managers will vary from practice to practice. In its broadest sense, the team role of practice manager can be described as follows.

The reception manager will be responsible for the running, design, and implementation of agreed administrative, financial, marketing, and personnel management systems on a continually developing basis, working as part of the practice team to assist in the provision of high-quality dental care services to our patients. The practice manager must further the practice's objectives for the provision of quality dental services in line with the practice's ethos and with GDC guidelines.

Financial Management
- Check invoices and pay minor creditors in line with company guidance.
- Liaise with the employer on salary enquiries.
- Supervise all practice banking procedures.
- Clarify terms of business to clients and thus reduce incidents of bad debt and failed appointments.
- Ensure that relevant payment claims are made and reconciled.
- Streamline processes and reduce the amount of clinical surgery time used for non-clinical tasks.

Personnel Management
- Assist with recruitment, training, and induction procedures.
- Encourage, motivate, and mentor staff in line with practice policy.
- Deploy staff, maintaining appropriate staffing levels in line with practice policy.
- Maintain records and report to the employer on staff sickness and holidays.
- Operate the staff discipline and grievance system.
- Maintain a team culture of respect and equitability.
- Organise and record staff training.
- Coordinate arrangements for staff appraisals.
- Organise and participate in staff meetings.

Practice Development
- Monitor the appointment books.
- Promote the image of the practice in ways consistent with practice policy.
- Monitor client feedback.
- Design administrative systems within the remit of your position.

- Maintain NHS and Independent/Dental Complaints Service (DCS) complaints procedures.
- Maintain the referrals system.
- Perform other related duties to maintain a high standard of patient care.
- Work with the lead dentists to monitor compliance with clinical governance consistent with practice guidelines.
- Oversee the implementation of the practice business and marketing plan.

General

- Arrange promotional events to raise the profile of the practice within the local community.
- Review and streamline procedures.
- Liaise with suppliers and representatives on behalf of the practice.
- Ensure compliance with health and safety legislation, the Disability Discrimination Act, and fire safety law.
- Oversee the maintenance of all practice equipment.
- Inspect all parts of the practice weekly; record and report deficiencies or malfunctions in line with practice policy.
- Supervise security of the building and alarm system and maintain a list of key holders.
- Maintain the first aid box, accident book, and other such compliance measures.

Patient Services

- Ensure the efficient operation of the patient recall system.
- Ensure the effective operation of patient complaints procedures.
- Respond to patient queries in a polite and professional manner.
- Ensure sufficient high-quality information is available for patients.

Reception Manager Personal Specifications

Essential Attributes

- Appropriate qualifications, fitness to practice certification, Criminal Records Bureau clearance.
- Computer literacy.
- Excellent communication skills.
- Customer interface experience.
- Proactive approach.
- Previous experience of working in a supervisory role within the health-care sector.
- 'Can do' attitude.

Desirable Attributes

- Recent experience of working within a team in a general dental practice.
- Experience of communicating nonclinical terms of dental care to colleagues and patients.
- Team player with strong relationship-building skills with colleagues and patients.

- Marketing or sales experience.
- Diligence.
- Motivation and keenness to further their professional development.

Salary

The practice manager role is still developing, as is the structure of the dental profession. With substantial changes in the business aspects of dentistry, the role of practice manager will continue to develop, offering managers a wide range of opportunities for personal and professional growth.

2

Administration

Alongside their customer care duties, receptionists are often responsible for the smooth running of the administrative systems that enable the clinical team to do their work. In this chapter, we will define those systems and consider how well they operate and how user-friendly they are in your practice.

The Administrative Role on the Front Desk

The receptionist is the crucial link between the public and the practice team. High-quality, consistent administrative services are, without exception, the result of clearly defined systems, backed up with training and resources for those operating those systems.

Methodical working systems portray an image of professionalism. Receptionists usually work under pressure, needing to multitask in a hectic environment. Nevertheless, working at an untidy desk, as shown in Figure 2.1, does not project the professional, everything's-under-control atmosphere that puts patients at ease. Receptionists need clear, structured working processes to avoid projecting an image that the practice is chaotic. Receptionist must learn to follow systems designed for working effectively under pressure.

Excellent receptionists learn to judge and respond to the moods of patients, dentists, and work colleagues. When practical and interpersonal skills are blended, the result is confident, competent receptionist services. The role of the reception supervisor it to apply practical skills in ways that support the development of those skills in the people whose work they supervise.

The familiar role of the nurse/receptionist has long been established in the dental sector.

In every business sector, the success is dependent on good operating systems. Computerisation enables dental practices to implement standard systems easily. Modern computers systems allow operators to access data and to analyse performance and relative costs. Many use computerised appointment books and, as a result, can investigate attendance and failure rates. They can produce accurate information about patient numbers and treatment uptake. Without this type of information, practice administration cannot accurately identify trends and plan timely responses.

Dental Reception and Supervisory Management, Second Edition. Glenys Bridges.
© 2019 John Wiley & Sons Ltd. Published 2019 by John Wiley & Sons Ltd.
Companion website: www.wiley.com/go/bridges/dental

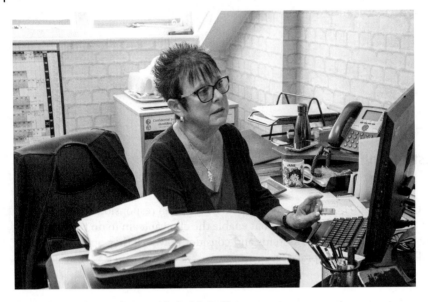

Figure 2.1 Working with an untidy desk is inefficient.

Building Dynamic Systems

Since the 1930s, the business world has been increasingly aware of the need for companies to 'do the right things, in the right ways. It is also aware that the needs of *purchasers*[1] and *providers*[2] change over time and that they need to develop administrative systems that keep up with these changing needs. Sometimes systems change over time in reaction to circumstances. If these unplanned changes are made without consideration of the bigger picture, systems become:

- Too complicated to run smoothly
- Inconsistent, or randomly applied
- Inefficient and ineffective because they duplicate work

Dental Reception Systems

Reception supervisors oversee a vast range of administration systems; these will typically include systems for patients, clinicians, operation management, and quality standards. The responsibilities under each area are described in the following.

Patients

- Appointments
- Recalls

---

1 Dental patients.
2 Dental teams.

- Collecting fees
- Information and education
- Records
- Medical histories
- Consent
- Communication

Clinicians

- Availability of materials
- Staff rotas
- Infection control
- Communication
- Lab work

Operations

- Accounts payable
- Banking
- Premises maintenance
- Health and Safety
- Telecommunications

Quality Standards

- Quality care regulations
- Information governance
- Standards for the dental team:
  - Confidentiality
  - Consent
  - Putting patients interests first
  - Safeguarding patient and office records

Keeping Systems Fit for Purpose

Quality administrative systems are effective, efficient, and continuously improving, as shown in Figure 2.2.

Effectiveness

Before you can assess how well an administration system works, it is necessary to define the results that the system should ideally achieve. Then performance can be measured against the 'ideal standard' – these measures are benchmarks or key performance

Name of System:		
Date:	**Rating**	**Reasons**
Effectiveness *The extent to which the system achieves its aims*		
Efficiency:	**Rating**	**Reasons**
Economy *How the system uses resources and materials*		
Adaptability *How the systems processes respond to the needs of users*		
User-friendliness *The user experience when working with the system*		
Reliability *Does the system produce consistent results*		
Action plan to increase quality ratings 1 2 3 4		

Figure 2.2 Quality audit.

indicators (KPI). Many systems will have more than one of these. A KPI for an appointment system might look like this:

> An appointment system should deliver a patient to the practice five minutes before the clinician is ready to treat them, to allow administrative processes to be completed and minimise the time the patient waits to see a dentist.

The extent to which a system delivers its KPIs defines the system's level of *effectiveness*. So, for example, if 80% of patients arrive and are seen on time for their appointments, then the effectiveness of the system can be rated as an 8. However, there are numerous reasons why systems do not meet their KPIs. It may be because that time allocation for each patient is unrealistic, and the clinicians must rush through the last patients of each session to finish on time (or not). Once the factual measures of effectiveness are determined, the next step is to understand the reasons for any underperformance and how to make improvements to increase the system's effectiveness.

Efficiency

Efficiency is a measure of *how* systems work. KPIs consider the following:

- *Economy.* Does the system make economical use of materials and time? Is it cost effective?
- *Adaptability.* If something unexpected happens, can the system deal with it? For example, can you see emergency patients without running late?
- *User friendliness.* Are team members trained to operate the system? What are the team members' experiences of the system? How do patients experience the system?
- *Reliability.* Does the system produce consistent results?

Continuous Improvement

The ratings from your audit show your system's current level of performance. If the performance is weak, you will be able to identify areas of weakness by the individual scores. To make targeted changes, it is a good idea to involve the users of the systems. Ask them for their ideas and feedback before deciding on what changes or adaptations to make.

When the ratings are good, do not rest on your laurels. Strive to continuously improve administrative systems. If you rate a 9, ask what it would take to be able to rate a 10. Then consider ways to add that additional point. Once the changes have been incorporated into the system and have had time to show their effects, reaudit to ensure that the increased quality in one area has not been at the cost of quality elsewhere in the system.

To analyse the quality of an administrative system:

1) Determine a rating for each of the factors listed in Figure 2.2 with a rating between 1 and 10 (with to be the ideal scenario in column 2 in Figure 2.2).
2) Give the reasons for the ratings given in column 3.
3) Add the numbers of the ratings and divide by 5 to get the overall picture of the quality of the system.
4) Suggest quality improvements.

Supervising Administrative Tasks Carried out by Receptionists in Your Practice

For logical reasons, many practices locate their receptionist desks by the front door and telephone. As a result, the reception area becomes a busy thoroughfare and not a suitable place to safeguard patient confidentiality, when discussing aspects of medical history, treatment requirements, or money. In some larger practices, this can be addressed by employing a care coordinator to address confidential administrative matters in a quieter area of the practice. This is a particularly effective way to address matters such as assisting patients to make applications for financing high-cost treatment plans.

Receptionists handle a vast range of administrative tasks. Some of these can be handled in the bustling reception area in the practice waiting room; others should be addressed in a private back office. Look at the following list of tasks below and identify the ideal place to deal with them:

- Customer care
- 'Meet and greet'
- Sale of sundry goods
- Highlighting the range of treatments available at the practice
- Medical history taking
- Confirming patients' details
- Answering patients' questions about treatment plans
- Answering telephones
- Handling money – cash or credit cards

Using the Practice Appointment Book

The appointment book is the most important tool for practices (see Figure 2.3). A well-run appointment book ensures:

- Steady patient flow ensures no excessive waiting for patients or clinicians.
- Clinicians have an interesting and varied working day.
- Equipment for each treatment is available when required.

Time Efficiency

To achieve these outcomes, receptionists must understand treatment room procedures. The practice needs to set booking rules for treatments and check-ups to make the best

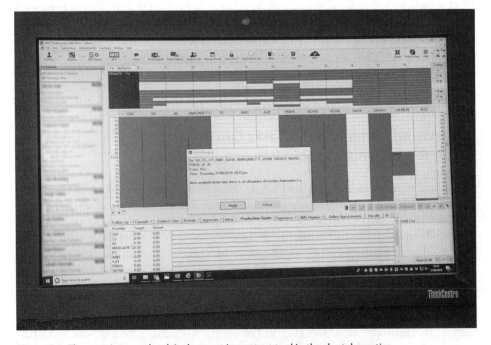

Figure 2.3 The appointment book is the most important tool in the dental practice.

use of the available appointment time, and the appointment book needs to be filled each day. This is where receptionists can make the most significant impact on the financial success of the practice. The appointment book can be used to monitor the following:

- Performance regarding seeing patients on time
- Ensuring appointments are available within a reasonable period
- Multiple appointments are well coordinated.

The practice's time is rationed through the appointment book, making it one of the most important time-management tools in practice.

Profitability

Pearly White Dental Care: Case Study 1

At Pearly White Dental Care, a single-handed dental practice, the appointment booking policy sets out appointments in 15-minute blocks.
Pearly White Dental Care needs to earn £400.00 per hour.
Treatment fees have been calculated as follows:

- Each 15-minute treatment generates £100.00.
- Practice is open 9 a.m.–1 p.m. and 2 p.m.–5 p.m. Monday to Friday (seven hours per day).

On this basis, the practice can offer 28 appointment blocks per day. Recently, the receptionist has stopped booking the 12.45 and 4.45 appointments each day as a precaution against the treatment sessions from running over into the lunch hour or past closing time.

Questions
1) What impact will this booking change have on practice income?
   - Per week
   - Per year (the practice works 48 weeks in a year)
2) What instructions would you give to a new receptionist to get the best results from your appointment book?

Rules for an Effective and Efficient Reception Desk

Figure 2.4 provides a table on the training needs for receptions to keep an efficient appointment book. Figure 2.5 discusses where various reception tasks should be carried out. The following steps will help keep an effective an efficient reception desk.

1) *Always keep accurate records.* Accurate patient records are basic requirements of good business. Clinical recordkeeping is taught in dental school. All too often, this learning is not carried over into practice administration. Clear recordkeeping systems create audit paths and are essential for good administration. Producing a reception manual and following its procedures in a disciplined way will ensure high-quality systems.
2) *Always pay attention to detail.* In a busy reception area, you will often be expected to work on more than one task at a time. If the pressure created by working in this way leads you to shortcut certain procedures, you will store up problems for the future.

Controlling the appointment book in your practice

Training needs for receptionists to control the appointment book

	Needs of the practice	Training aims and objectives
Patient satisfaction		
Workflow management		
Managing cash flow		
Essential aspects of time management		

Figure 2.4 Training receptionists to keep an efficient appointment book.

Activity Chapter 2 Fig 3		
Discuss where various reception tasks should be carried out. Give reasons for chosen locations		
Reception task	Why on the front desk	Why not on the front desk
Cashing up		
Correspondence		
Accounts		
Medical history		
Explaining treatment plans		

Figure 2.5 Where reception tasks should be performed.

By skimming over the details of tasks such as calculating patient charges, you create extra work for yourself and undermine the professionalism of the practice.

3) *Always keep your working area tidy*. A tidy desk portrays an orderly mind.

4) *Always follow procedures*. The best way to create an atmosphere of professionalism is to follow the tried and tested procedures, which have been proven to produce satisfactory results.

5) *Always watch for changing needs*. Just because a system is working well at the moment does not mean that it will work well forever. Good systems adapt to meet changing needs. This does not mean that systems can be changed on a whim. All changes should be made in consultation with the system's users and should be well communicated and documented.

6) *Always measure results*. If you receive a complaint, you know something is not to the patient's liking, but there is evidence that even when they're not happy, many patients do not complain to you. However, they do grumble to anyone else who will listen. Always invite feedback from patients. Listen to patients talking to each other in the waiting room and then make improvements based on their comments.

7) *Never overcomplicate tasks*. It is not a good idea to make practice administration any more complicated than it needs to be. Overcomplicated systems lead to mistakes and omissions.

8) *Never try to be all things to all people*. It is commendable to aim to please patients and colleagues alike. However, you can end up pleasing nobody if you are shortcutting procedures and making changes to please one person at the expense of others. The art is to know just how flexible you can be without creating situations in which you please nobody.

9) *Never run out of stock materials*. Running out of the material that you require to do your work is just bad organisation. Always keep stock levels to hand, which will enable you to work smoothly and professionally.

10) *Never jump from job to job, leaving loose ends*. Working on a busy reception desk can mean you need to jump from job to job without finishing any of them. Make sure that you return to all of your loose ends and complete tasks so that they cannot bring about nasty shocks in the future.

Providing Written Instructions

The role of a reception supervisor is to enable the staff they supervise to work to the best of their ability. They aim to develop reliable quality systems. Standardising processes ensures the reliability of administration systems.

How to Produce Reception Working Instructions

Clear working instructions help the reader to accomplish tasks efficiently and successfully. They form a vital part of your reception manual. To produce working instructions, follow the steps described in these sections.

First, select a reception task and observe the task being performed. Note the individual actions being undertaken. If you would like anyone doing that job to replicate that way of working, create written instructions that map those actions. However, if there are parts of their approach that can be improved, this is your chance to reshape how the task is performed in the future.

When Drafting Your Instructions

- Limit each step to one idea.
- Keep the sentences simple.
- Begin each sentence with a verb, e.g. **Open** the folder.
- Include diagrams or pictures wherever appropriate.
- Ensure the steps follow the most efficient sequence.
- Use the KISS principle – Keep It Simple, Stupid.

Testing and Re-Drafting

- Observe someone who is not familiar with the task trying out your instructions.
- Note any difficulties the person has in following the instructions.
- Revise your instructions.
- Observe someone else performing the task to your instructions.
- Repeat this process until the task is performed without difficulty.

Tasks done according to clear instructions are performed the same way each time. Also, activities are performed in the same order, irrespective of who performs the task. This level of standardisation can only be achieved through the development and distribution of standard working procedures. These will usually be part of a procedures manual.

3

Marketing

No other member of the dental team has more opportunities to gain insights into patients' needs and wants than the receptionist. The front-of-house role allows team members to spend time talking to and listening to patients (see Figure 3.1). In this unit, you will discover a range of ways to turn those patient interactions into marketing opportunities for the benefit of the patients, dental team and the dental business.

Marketing Definition

> *Marketing is defined as creating, communicating and delivering goods and services which have value for patients, colleagues and society?*
>
> Marketing is the process by which dental businesses can create value for patients and build strong patient relationships and ongoing patient loyalty.
>
> Marketing is about creating value, solutions and relationships.
>
> Marketing skills include sales techniques, communication to build patient relationships and creating value, for patients and the dental team.

Marketing aims to do the following:

- Identify patients' profiles and dental needs.
- Satisfy the needs of patient groups.
- Win patients' ongoing loyalty.

The term *marketing* developed from an original meaning, which literally referred to going to a market to buy or sell goods or services. Marketing aims to establish ways to ensure that the needs of patients are recognized and fully met, this begins with:

- Effective market research
- Skilful evaluation of findings

Success in marketing requires a good grasp of your patients' psychologies, to understand the impact of emotional and financial factors on their purchasing behaviour.

Dental Reception and Supervisory Management, Second Edition. Glenys Bridges.
© 2019 John Wiley & Sons Ltd. Published 2019 by John Wiley & Sons Ltd.
Companion website: www.wiley.com/go/bridges/dental

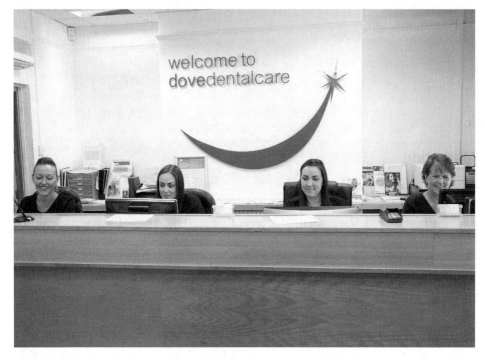

Figure 3.1 The receptionists have opportunities to gain insights into patients' needs and wants.

Market Research

When conducting market research, always consider your patients' rights and ensure all activities meet appropriate legal, cultural, ethical, and environmental standards for dental businesses. Successful marketing begins with a clear idea of what you want to achieve, such as:

- Better patient retention
- A raised public profile
- Increased referrals
- A reduction in fail to attends

Market research is the beginning point when the practice:

- Wants to explore a marketing idea
- Wants to find the best way to increase turnover

When researching, it is a mistake to be so focused on the original idea that you overlook alternative courses of action would be more productive.

Marketing Mix

The marketing mix is a technique used to identify the best way to bring products and services to the market. The most successful businesses are built around understanding and meeting their patients' requirements.

Focusing on patients increases the chances of competitive success; basing a range of business activities on the marketing mix can do this. In this way, decisions are made with the aim of creating 'best-fit' solutions to meet the recognized needs and wants of the dental team (providers of services) and the patients (purchasers of dental services).

When this balance is right, it will influence patients' perceptions of the practice and therefore their motivation and purchasing behaviour. Neil Borden first introduced the marketing mix theory in 1953, in his presidential address to the American Marketing Association when he coined the term *marketing mix*. Prominent marketer E. Jerome McCarthy proposed the 5P classification in 1960, which has seen numerous variations on the theme, dependent on sector requirements.

One expansion of McCarthy's classification system includes these factors in arriving at the right marketing mix for a business:

- Price
- Promotion
- Place
- Product
- People

Price

Price is a critical element of the mix, which can become a deal breaker. Patients will always look for value for money. The challenge in marketing is to convince patients that the features and benefits of the product are excellent value for money. It is widely considered that patients buy the *benefits* derived from their purchases, although the *features* of the purchase will influence the decision as to which product to buy:

- *Features* of treatments are the specifications of treatment, which may include convenient appointment times, limited time in the chair, and interest-free finance availability.
- *Benefits* of treatments are that they may be able to eat, speak, and smile with more confidence.

An essential aspect of the cost is the ability of the patient to understand the benefits in conjunction with the price. This understanding has the potential to shift the patient's focus away from the cost to the value of treatment.

When pricing services and treatments it is vital to calculate the *cost of sales*. In this way, you ensure the price is viable. When businesses price goods and services to beat their competitors on price alone, they risk underpricing and financial ruin.

Promotion

Promotional aspects include anything that affects the practice image. It includes features such as advertising, direct marketing, packaging, personal selling, public relations, and sales promotions.

Advertising to raise awareness and promote services can be very costly unless you make use of a range of ways to advertise free of charge. There are plenty of places to get your practice mentioned for nothing, such as local papers and consumer information guides. There is an increasing number of web directories now, which carry free listings. On the old-fashioned side of things, stick your leaflets on free notice boards in libraries, halls, and community centres, medical practices, and staff rooms.

The media can be a significant source of free publicity that can give your practice an enormous boost. New products or features in the national, even local, newspapers can bring in millions of pounds. A quarter-page advertisement in the nationals would cost you thousands while the equivalent in editorial space is free! You can email details of a new practice or innovative procedure to the editorial desk of your chosen publication and take it from there.

Keep your website up to date; ensure you include details of all existing and evolving products and services. Be aware of keywords used by Internet search engines – make sure you use words on your website that prospective patients will use when searching for dental services.

Word of mouth is a primary source of new patients, so give it a helping hand by giving patients a simple referral form and offer them incentives to introduce a friend to your products. People like to know about how your existing patients feel about the practice, so put 'thank you' letters and other positive publicity – press features, etc. – in your brochures and on your website.

Becoming high profile in the local community is an excellent way to attract attention. Being a sponsor can often yield significant publicity for a modest investment. Typical examples are amateur or professional football clubs (you can pay for the kit and put your name on the shirts), arts organizations, community groups, and charity fundraising events.

Place

Place includes the features of your practice premises. This is an important part of the marketing mix, as is the availability of car parking or public transport.

Consider the profile of the patients you want to attract. If you are aiming to be a family practice, including child-friendly aspects of the practice will make you attractive to families, whereas if you are in an area with large numbers of industrial or commercial units, you may want to make adults the focus of your patient base. Decisions about the features of your premises should be made with consideration of the people directly or indirectly involved in the delivery and consumption of your product, including the dental team. Their interactions can influence the perceived value of your product and organization.

Product

When considering your product, rather than focusing on the features of treatments, look at the benefits you are selling to your patients, as this is what interests them. Present products in ways that show you understand your patients' requirements. Design services to satisfy patients' consumer needs and continually fine-tune products to accommodate changing needs and market conditions.

People

The socioeconomic status of the area in which your practice is located will be a factor in the type of patients you attract. Whatever their social status, some patient behaviours are always undesirable:

- Being rude or aggressive to the team
- Failing to keep appointments
- Not paying for treatments

The practice should have clear policies and requirements that patients are aware of to establish the practice's stipulations for patient behaviour.

If you practice in a town centre, then you may want to design and promote an image of your practice to attract workers, rather than families. If your practice is in a suburb, you may prefer to project a child-friendly image. Carefully name the practice to make it clear what your ideal patient group is, e.g. The Family Dental Care Centre.

Effective Marketing to Create a Competitive Edge

The most successful practices do something better than their competitors. There are many ways to create a competitive edge. The best place to begin this is to recognize and value your patients' needs. For example, high-tech, state-of-the-art practices will appeal to some patients, whereas others prefer features that make the practice more friendly and homely.

To create a competitive edge requires attention to quality aspects of your service, in particular:

- Quality of service
- Quality of products

Your patients will experience this as flexibility and service.

Flexibility

As a small business, you can offer more flexible services than large companies. This flexibility can enable you to meet patients' individual needs. You can also provide specialized pre- or post-treatment services that enhance the patient care offered.

Service

Knowing your patients and taking an interest in them as people is an essential way of building respect between the practice and patients. Finding ways to make patients feel valued will develop your competitive edge.

Product Sales

When patients have seen their dentist and hygienist, their oral health and home care routines are at the forefront of their minds. Therefore, this is the perfect time for them to stock up on the products that clinicians recommend. Some specialized products are not readily available in local stores, which offers the dental practice an opportunity to provide patients with a service they need and make a legitimate profit.

Most practices have a skills gap when it comes to the presentation and sale of retail goods. It is time that dental teams became more switched on to the potential of retail to offer benefits to patients and the dental business. At present, most retail goods are placed behind the desk or in a glass display case. What's more, there are no prices shown, either! Patients might be willing to purchase a product without actually touching it, as they do online, but they are unlikely to show great interest in a product for which both product and price are masked. The result of this style of retailing is a massive loss of revenue for the practice. It can give patients the impression that they are creating extra work for the hard-pushed receptionists by asking about the products they want to buy, so they might prefer to just leave and spend £20.00 in the local supermarket!

If we take the average dental practice with 3000 patients, visiting twice a year plus, it is reasonable to assume that 10 000 visits will be made to reception on any given year. Let's assume with skilful displays of product and prompting from the oral health practitioners that the average patient was to spend £5.00 a visit. By the end of the year, sales will add up to £50 000. Estimating a typical 50% markup, that is a potential £12 500 to the bottom line of the practice income.

So, what can the receptionist do to make this scenario more likely?

1) Put items within reach of the patients to stimulate the 'impulse buy' instinct.
2) Make the prices visible – people base their purchasing decisions on cost.
3) Start to help patients with their purchases. When you are buying clothes or shoes, how often do you choose to accessorize your purchases with the products presented at the pay points?

Although the sale of home care products in dental practices are secondary purchases when patients are purchasing products recommended by their dentist or hygienist for better home care and long-term oral health, ensure that ethical selling is the underpinning approach to retailing goods. The guiding principle is to make the recommended products easily accessible, and sell only what is recommended by appropriately qualified dental professionals.

Retail is not a dirty word in dentistry. It is quite simply a logical extension of the practice's care for its patients. Dentists need to provide what patients want in a clear and easily accessible way.

Dental Products as a Patient Service

Not only have dental practices discovered the value of selling home care products, but also patients have come to value buying products in the reception area of their chosen dental practice. Today the provision of dental products for sale in practices is viewed as being a service to patients. Nevertheless, there are several factors that reception staff should be aware of, to meet the best interests of both the practice and patients when selling dental goods to patients.

The professional status of dentists means that they have a duty of care to ensure, as far as possible, that the products they sell to their patients are scientifically proven to be safe and suitable for the patients that buy them. Dentists have a responsibility to research all products they endorse by selling or recommending to their patients. They must ensure that all necessary information is passed on to patients so that they can make informed decisions at the point of sale.

Some patients will need specialist home care products, such as orthodontic brushes, which are not always available at the supermarket. Practices offer a great convenience to their patients by making these products available at the office.

By offering products for sale, you are ensuring that the recommended products are available, which makes it less likely that patients will opt for substitutes that are readily accessible, familiar, or cheaper and less effective. The range of dental home care products available in the average supermarket is vast. How can patients make the right choice when selecting products? We can only be sure that patients are purchasing products suited to their dental needs by offering products and supporting them to make informed choices.

As dental practices are businesses, the profits from the sale of goods are a consideration. The level of sales and profit margins from sales vary vastly from practice to practice. At the very least, it is important to cover the costs of purchasing the goods, product promotions, displays, and managing the stock. These aspects of product sales, which are often the responsibility of the reception team or the care coordinator, require the development of a range of retail skills to perform these tasks well. The next sections address some of these factors.

Purchasing

Purchasing is more than buying – it includes identifying trends and fashions so that you can buy goods to interest the consumers. It is a good idea to keep an eye open for the big company advertising campaigns in the media, so that you can benefit from their advertising expenditure, offering goods that have already been heavily sold to patients by the manufacturer. You should also keep records of what sells and when, so that you can prepare for any seasonal trends. Storage space can be a problem in some practices; make sure products are suitably stored.

Product Promotion

You need to let patients know about the range of products you sell, and make them easy for patients to buy. It is a good idea to make information on the products available and to ask patients if they would like to buy products. This means that receptionists need to be well informed about the features and benefits of each product – yes, even the toothbrushes.

Displays

The presentation is very influential. Do not be tempted to put all your stock on view; make an eye-catching display such as in Figure 3.2, showing each product marked with its price, giving a professional feel to your sales effort. The days are gone when you can place a mug stuffed with toothbrushes for sale on the reception desk.

The receptionist plays just as important a role as any of the other members of the dental team. With the knowledge that is at hand, the receptionist very often answers patients' queries, either face-to-face or by telephone. These could include, for example, which toothbrush is best for a young child or a child undergoing orthodontic treatment, or which toothpaste is best, one with fluoride or without.

Be open to listening as the patient asks about various products. Maybe the patient is talking about toothbrushes but is really wondering whether to make an appointment about a lump or rough patch inside his, or her mouth. The receptionist who is attentive and has at hand the current dental health information can make the patient feels comfortable with the more urgent queries and can advise the patient in such a way as to not cause alarm and at the same time ensure that the patient receives prompt and professional care.

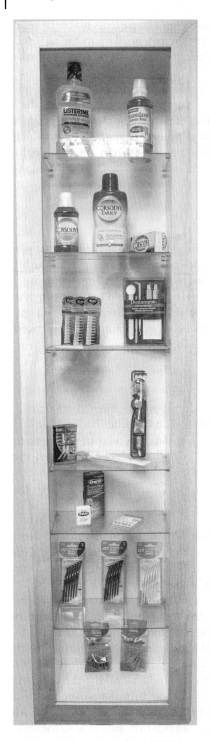

Figure 3.2 Create an eye-catching display for products sold to patients.

4

Financial Administration

Financial Aspects of Patient Consent

As dental practices align with other small businesses and delegate aspects of cash management to senior staff, reception teams need a new range of financial management skills. A new generation of delegated work requires input from reception leaders able to set budgets, oversee management accounts, and forecast expected expenditure (expenses) and the fees generation (revenue) on a month-by-month basis.

Management accounts organise income and expenditure into categories or activities (e.g. telephone costs, sundries, materials, etc.). Forecasted activity is then monitored to identify whether year-to-date finances are running to plan.

Managing Cash Flow

The reception team need to govern cash flow – the overall purpose of cash flow management is to make sure there is enough cash available to run the practice. Businesses can manage cash flow by comparing a cash flow statement to a cash flow projection, which should be part of the business plan. Cash flow relates to the actual cash transactions. It is recorded in the cash book, which is the primary means of tracking cash and recording income and expenditure.

Credit and Collections

To maintain a healthy cash flow, the reception team needs to create guidelines for collecting fees. Receptionists need to work closely with managers to set out and implement the terms and conditions of business and also the circumstances under which credit is extended to patients.

Protecting Practice Income

Ensuring that all treatment fees earned are collected, accounted for, and banked is the essence of good cash flow. To ensure that the correct fees are collected, on time from each patient requires a wide span of reception skills.

Dental Reception and Supervisory Management, Second Edition. Glenys Bridges.
© 2019 John Wiley & Sons Ltd. Published 2019 by John Wiley & Sons Ltd.
Companion website: www.wiley.com/go/bridges/dental

Communication Skills

Patient's fees can amount to significant sums of money. When patients only consider the amount they are paying for their dental procedures, rather than the benefits they will gain from that treatment, some believe that the charges are excessive. For many people, money is a sensitive issue. In times of financial downturn, this can only worsen.

It is the role of the dentist to explain treatments and costs to their patients. However, we know from experience that many patients will then go on to ask the receptionist for further explanations about treatments, costs, and payment options.

When discussing financial aspects of their care, some patients feel uncomfortable if others can overhear and their confidentiality is not respected. When designing reception areas, it is essential to include somewhere to talk in privacy about payment options or other issues.

Administration Skills

Accurately calculating treatment fees for the first time every time is an essential financial skill for dental receptionists. It is not surprising that patients get very annoyed when they pay the price requested for their treatment, only to be asked for more money at a future date because the price was not correctly calculated.

Patients also become irritated when they have paid their treatment fees, but because it was not correctly recorded a repeated request for payment is made. These and all other administration errors are avoided when clear protocols and procedures for collecting and recording patient payments are in place.

Annoying patients because of errors and omissions are to be avoided, but so, too, is the error of failing to collect patient's fees that are due. Patients who miss appointments are a drain on the practice's resources and ability to earn money. Far worse is when the practice had borne the cost of providing a patient's treatment but has not been paid.

Accurately operating clear, straightforward accounting procedures is a primary skill for dental receptionists. The practice must set policy for patient payment, and the reception team need must consistently follow them.

Terms of Business

Almost every successful business transaction requires an explicit understanding between the purchaser and the provider. It is essential to clarify each party's expectations and the terms of business, including when, where, and by whom services will be provided. Any businesses that do not specify their terms of business with patients leave themselves open to disputes and misunderstandings. Agreed terms of business are a sound basis for building respectful relationships between purchasers and providers. Terms of business specify points such as the following:

- Appointments available
- Cancellation requirements
- When fees are due
- Payment requirements
- Payment in instalments

- Responsibilities and liabilities if the patient fails to complete a course of treatment
- What happens if the practice needs to cancel an appointment
- The practice fairness and equality policy
- The practice complaints procedures

   Patients should be asked to read and sign this copy of the practice terms and conditions

Informing Patients of Fees and Payment Terms

Patients complain when their expectations of good service have not been met. Most dental complaints are about nonclinical aspects of their care. These issues arise when a patient's expectations have not been met, and there has been a communication breakdown. When communication breaks down, one of the most serious consequences is a loss of informed consent. The patient consents to be treated and agrees to pay the fees associated with their treatment plan.

   Informed consent applies when a person can be said to have given consent based on his or her understanding of the facts, and the implications and consequences of an action. The law necessitates that before any health care professional can examine or treat a patient, fully informed consent must be obtained.

   Consent can be either:

- *Explicit* (specific consent to carry out a particular action)
- *Implied* (not expressly given by a patient, but inferred from their actions, the facts and circumstances of a situation, and sometimes a patient's silence or inaction)

   A signed estimate provides evidence that some discussion about the fees has taken place. This must be supported by an outline of the conversation, recorded in the patient's notes.

Written Estimates

Most receptionists will have at some time encountered a situation in which a treatment fee is due, but when a patient is asked to settle her account, she is shocked at the amount owed. At such times there are numerous issues of informed consent and patients' rights that have been infringed. How can patients have consented if they are not aware of the full facts?

   The patient should be provided with a written estimate specifying the following:

- Treatment prescribed
- Treatment fees
- Appointments needed to complete the course of treatment
- Appointment availability

   Only when they have the full facts can an informed choice be made. When receptionists can take the time with patients to explain their estimate and map their appointments, patients feel better cared for, and so are more likely to keep their appointments, turn up on time, and pay their bill.

Payments Due

For many people, money is the most critical factor in the decision to purchase dental treatment. Irrespective of their financial circumstances, people attach vital importance to the cost of dental care. Therefore, it is essential to take a sensitive approach when discussing fees and to clarify payment terms, essentially communicating the rights and responsibilities of both parties.

The practice has a responsibility to be clear and straightforward about treatment costs and about practice policy on collecting fees. Ambiguous or inconsistent information regarding the payments are the most significant single causes of bad debts and complaints. To avoid misunderstandings or ambiguity, receptionists should not only be sensitive to patients' concerns, but they must also avoid falling into the trap of making assumptions about whether patients can afford treatments prescribed for them.

Here are some practical tips for collecting fees:

- Be firm but not aggressive when requesting payment from patients.
- Be sensitive to patients' needs for privacy.
- Use plain, old-fashioned manners; don't forget to say *please* and *thank you*.
- Be clear and give adequate details on costs and when payment is required.
- Avoid nasty surprises by providing written estimates.
- Offer clear, written details about *methods* of payment.
- Ask patients *how* they wish to pay.
- Emphasize value, not cost.

Collecting Fees Patient Payments

The clear majority of receptionists are engaged and enthusiastic about their role in patient care. There is often less clarity about their role as the practice's financial regulator, the person responsible for ensuring the money owed to the practice for treatments is collected on time, and or implementing the practice's policy for managing patient's fees. Besides collecting fees, receptionists are also responsible for the safekeeping of cash on the premises.

As already noted, while patients who consistently fail to keep appointments drain practice resources, the worst type of patients are those who attend, have their treatment, and leave without paying. At best they create unnecessary work chasing bad debt; at worst they are a threat to the viability of the practice.

Informing Patients of Fees Due

A friendly assertive approach works best where payments requests are concerned. Communication is the cornerstone of active fee collection. Written estimates are the payment contract between the patient and the practice. Even when patients are in breach of contract, avoid taking a confrontational stance, especially in public areas of the practice; instead, offer a private talk with the practice manager. Payments not collected become bad debts, which must be carefully monitored and pursued efficiently and professionally. Ideally there should be no bad debts, but in reality, this is not always achievable.

If bad debts have been a problem in the past, the introduction of a clear policy, consistently followed, usually reduces bad debts dramatically. Before any dental receptionist can excel as a financial regulator, management measures must be introduced to provide a clear framework of practice policies for all cash flow activities.

For example, practice policy for collecting patient's payments may say:

> It is our policy to provide patients with a written estimate and treatment plan, which they are required to sign to indicate their acceptance of the treatment plan and payment conditions before any treatment is undertaken.

Our policy is that:

- Patients are required to pay at each visit for the treatment carried out.
- All new patients are required to pay £** in advance at their first appointment.
- We reserve the right to ask any patient to pay for their treatment in advance.
- A 50% deposit is required when booking treatments exceeding £**.
- No further appointments can be booked for patients with overdue fees.
- Cancellations with less than 48 hours' notice and for missed appointments are charged at £10 for every 10 minutes booked; these fees will be classed as an outstanding balance.
- Fees can be paid by cash, cheque, credit, or debit card.

Unpaid fees will be subject to a 2% administration charge, and possible court action for collection.

Website

The practice image can be significantly enhanced when you have a website, designed to suit the needs of your patients. Your website is a place your patients can visit in their own time, to get to know the practice. Make sure your site offers a wide range of information about treatments, so that patient can see how you are working with them to maintain their oral well-being.

Perception of Value: Car Parking Issues and Welcome Packs

Patient attendance levels and cash flow are directly interlinked. Even when patients intend to keep their appointments, if they arrive at the location of the practice and cannot find a parking place, they are likely to go home again without attending.

If parking is a problem around your practice, it is advisable to let people know that additional time for parking will be required. If feasible, give details of public transport options, on the practice website, or in your welcome pack.

Patients' perceptions of *value* are directly linked to how *valued* they feel. Where patients' experiences at the practice are positive, they are more likely to recognise the value, rather than the cost, of treatment.

Research shows there to be a direct correlation between the quality of the relationship between practices and their patients and levels of unpaid accounts. Where the connections are respectful, there is less bad debt. The customer care advantages gained by providing a *welcome pack* to patients, to introduce the practices' team and ensure services are fully understood, will promote the perception of value and openness.

5

Staff Selection

One of the most significant difficulties facing dental businesses today is how to recruit high-quality people. How do you find the right calibre of staff? Over the past 10 years, the employment market, has been developing attractive packages for 'the right people'. In general, the dental market, however, has offered poor wages, no career structure, no pension schemes, and no fringe benefits. Is it any wonder that teachers and careers advisors actively discourage keen and bright youngsters when they ask about dental nursing as a career?

So how can a dental business compete in the job market with companies that have personnel departments, full of experts on all aspects of people management? The answer is, regularly spend a little time working *on* your business. In this way, you will get added value from the time spent working *in* your business. Working on your business means spending time deciding *what* you want to achieve and planning *how* to make it happen. Managers must identify the contributions needed from each member of the team. Having determined what you need from the team, you can create job descriptions and person specification. It's hardly rocket science, and job descriptions will be remarkably similar in many practices.

Dental professionals increasingly recognise that the key to building a focused, motivated and lasting team lies in doing the right things for existing employees. This attitude has its merits, although its most significant weakness lies in its assumption that we can change people to meet practice requirements.

Team spirit is severely damaged when a trusted colleague leaves the team. When selecting replacement staff, besides looking for skills and qualifications, also look for the characteristics suited to your practice's existing team – someone who will fit in

Research carried out by Development Dimensions International (2007) identified the 'career battery', a low-cost and highly effective tool to unearth qualities in individuals likely to lead to long-term service with their employer:

- Adaptability
- Passion for work
- Emotional maturity
- Positive disposition
- Self-efficacy

Dental Reception and Supervisory Management, Second Edition. Glenys Bridges.
© 2019 John Wiley & Sons Ltd. Published 2019 by John Wiley & Sons Ltd.
Companion website: www.wiley.com/go/bridges/dental

Building a lasting team is best achieved by selecting the right people in the beginning, since it is more realistic to select the right people to employ than to change the wrong applicants into the right employees.

The opinions of human resources experts on how to build a settled team differ: some suggest that selecting the right people requires anything from a clear view of what the practice needs and human nature – to a crystal ball! Many practice managers don't have a crystal ball, or the chance to use their staff section skills often enough to hone them into a fine art.

To screen applicants in favour of the required qualities, ask how they would react in certain situations or ask them to rate various actions in respect of their desirability for accomplishing goals.

Check for a 'job fit' by asks existing job holders to identify the critical characteristics of the role to be filled. During the interview, ask the candidate to discuss the features of their ideal job; the higher the correlation, the more likely that the candidate will not only be able to do the job but will be happy doing it in the long term.

Be clear about the level of commitment you require from your staff over and above the ability to fulfil the primary work role. You need the dental professionals on your team to take responsibility for maintaining their professional status and participate in Continuous Professional Development activities. Make this clear at the interview; specify the level of commitment required in the person specification and terms of employment.

Seek emotional maturity – the attributes of 'emotional maturity', and 'positive disposition' are crucial for health care workers. These attributes underpin customer care skills.

Research shows workers with these qualities display fewer negative work behaviours such as time-wasting or even theft. To select applicants with these qualities the interview process needs to search for examples of outstanding teamwork, customer focus and an ability to accomplish agreed goals.

Finding a candidate with the right approach to their personal and professional development is like finding the caterpillar that turns into a butterfly, rather than the moth that eats away at the fabric of your practice. Look for applicants with the desire to learn and develop, from success and the courage to learn from mistakes and setbacks.

Creating a work environment in which people want to stay long term is dependent upon recognising and balancing the needs of individuals with those of the dental business. Since those needs are constantly changing, it is essential that once you have found high-quality staff with the right attributes for long-term engagement, the practice shows the same sort of commitment to them as it expects from them.

Active recruitment includes processes for attracting, screening, and selecting the right people for a job. Building the right team will distinguish you from your competition. This unit will take you through the following seven necessary steps for recruitment:

1) Define the current needs of the practice, including the job and personal specifications.
2) Advertise.
3) Prepare a fulfilment pack and post the job.
4) Create a shortlist.
5) Interview.
6) Make the job offer.

Define the Current Needs of the Practice

Perfect Preparation Prevents Poor Performance

Recruitment policy and procedures should be a matter of record, ready to be used as and when required. Workforce planning begins with an organisational chart (see Figure 5.1), in which you produce a visual display of the practice and where each team member fits into the organisation.

The policy should cover:

- Where advertisements are placed and by whom
- Who interviews
- When interviews will be held
- Recordkeeping

Staffing Ratios

It is a mistake to replace staff like with like if the interests of the practice can be better served by bringing in new skills sets or employing someone to work different hours than those of the person who has left. Always have a current organisational chart to hand when making staffing decisions.

The formula for calculating the optimum staff ratio of 1.8 support staff for each full-time clinician is shown in Figure 5.2.

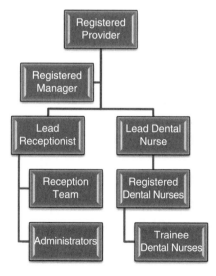

Figure 5.1 Organizational chart identifying the current needs of the practice.

Current staffing needs of the practice

Staffing Ratios

1   **Specify dentist hours by adding the hours for each dentist together**

Dentists	Hours
1	
2	
3	
4	
Total Hours	(A)

Dental Care Professional	Hours
1	
2	
3	
4	
Total Hours	(B)

Office Staff	Hours
1	
2	
3	
4	
Total Hours	(C)

Practice Manager Hours	(D)

Total Hours (B) + (C) + (D) =	(E)

Figure 5.2 Staffing ratios.

Job and Person Specifications

At the application stage, all applicants should receive the *job description* and *person specification* for the position that the applicant is seeking. The job description contains the following:

- General information about the practice and the job
- The primary purpose of the position
- List duties and tasks
- State working locations and conditions
- Reporting structures
- Salary rate

The person specification describes the ideal person for the job. It is a combination of physical, psychological, and experiential factors. Applicants' qualities should be assessed based on qualities such as the following:

1	Skills	Training, qualification, experience, and knowledge
2	Responsibility	Reliability, leadership, and sociability
3	Personality	Intelligence, judgement, maturity
4	Physical	Agility, stamina, special sensory requirements

Each of these qualities is classified as either essential or desirable. The desirable characteristics are then scored at the interview stage. Staff selection is a social science based on both policy and procedures and intuition.

The job description and person specification should be one document, which will support an equal-opportunity approach throughout the selection process, as each applicant has the same set of criteria to meet.

Staff selection is a matching process in which the manager needs to calculate the hard and soft factors to find the best fit for the position being filled. When an applicant expresses an interest in joining your team, the practice's first response should be to provide the job description and person-specific qualifications to be used in the staff selection process.

When preparing a job description, the inclusion of the phrase 'carry out other reasonable work-related tasks on request of the practice principal or practice manager' will eliminate the chances of staff adopting an 'It's not in my job description' attitude to nonroutine tasks.

Salary Considerations

Remunerate your team fairly; but don't pay more than the business can afford:

- Plan your staff remuneration budget.
- Consider offering results based bonuses.
- Reward loyalty.
- Set out a clear staff progression plans.

Staff salaries constitute a significant outlay for dental businesses. They are also one of the most common reasons for staff discontentment. When there are no clear criteria for calculating salaries, then it is likely that there will be a disparity leading to conflict or demotivation within the team.

Decide on a pay scale that rewards what you value the most, such as loyalty, added skills and qualifications, and performance, then apply this across the board. In theory, all payments will relate to a salary formula and so will not a cause of competition between team members.

Many staff employed in dental businesses work without any clear idea of what their employer expects from them. In short, they do not have a detailed job description and have never discussed with their employers, precisely what contribution they are supposed to make to the smooth running of the practice. Although most dental staff have a job description, It is calculated that as few as 20% of dental employers have discussed, specific work roles with their team.

When on the surface of things, all is well, and the practice is operating like a well-oiled machine, the idea of spending time and energy into a seemingly unnecessary task is not particularly attractive. Couple this with concerns that with a job description in place, individual members of staff could respond to requests to perform any additional duties by saying 'It's not in my job description!' and the idea of formalising job descriptions seem unattractive. Be assured that having explicit agreements with each member of the team is an investment is a fair, equal, and diverse workplace.

Personnel management activities are a support activity often sidelined in favour of 'core' activities. In dental practices, this is a legacy from the past when many dental teams comprised of the dentist and a nurse-receptionist. The dentist performed the dentistry, and the nurse-receptionist did what as they were told, under the direct supervision of the employing dentist, this approach suited to the micro-workplace environment and each person understood what was expected of him or her. All communication was verbal. Basic good manners were enough to keep things ticking over. As practices become larger and are more regulated, a more structured approach is essential.

Advertising Job Openings

Consideration of how to advertise situations available should be based on results of previous recruitment processes. It's essential to keep detailed records of your recruitment campaigns and evaluate their results for future reference.

Before deciding how to recruit for a position, think about:

- *What are your first impressions?* The recruitment initiative should give you an opportunity to get a feel for the person.
- How will you stand out from other employers? Be creative in your campaign.
- *How do big organisations recruit?* Observe how they attract recruits – they pay a lot of money to maintain a human resource department; you might be able to apply some of their expertise to your own operation.
- *Is your advertisement accurate?* Show the skills desired and salary scale offered. Otherwise, you may waste time interviewing over/underqualified applicants or outstanding applicants that you cannot afford.

Preparing a Fulfilment Pack and Posting the Job

Relying on a brief conversation over the telephone could potentially lead to wasted time, so prepare a fulfilment pack containing:

- Application form
- Information about the practice
- Job description and person specification
- Details about the closing date for applications and the proposed time for interviews

The pack can be in paper or electronic format. There are many options for posting jobs online now. However, ensure that before you and the applicant invest any more time in taking the application any further, the terms and expectations of the position are well communicated. Asking for an application form is much better than requesting just a resumé or curriculum vitae (CV) because it will standardise the information gathered, assisting you in making fair decisions about whom to invite to an interview.

Creating the Shortlist

It will be easier to shortlist – i.e. narrow down your candidates – if you use the same categories of information to assess each applicant:

- Look at all the resumé's together.
- Grade them in order of best liked to least liked (identify where they are going to add value to your practice).

- Determine if you can tell if they have researched your practice.
- Shortlist candidates to no more than 5–6 people to interview.
- Send a letter to the unsuccessful candidates as a matter of courtesy.
- Create an interview record sheet in preparation for the first interview.

Upon return of the application form, you can score applicants against the person specification details and select for interviews. Standardised letters should be in place to notify anyone not selected for an interview.

Interviewing

Always give at least one week's notice when scheduling the interview appointment. Create an interview schedule allowing equal and ample time for each applicant. Allow for delays and time for the panel to discuss applications directly after the interview.

When selecting staff, be aware that you cannot expect to change the person you employ. You can train the person, but you cannot fundamentally change their personality. Look at the outward signs of their character observable in their appearance – are they clean, tidy, well groomed? If these factors are important to you, they should be included and scaled on the interview record form. See Appendix 5.1 for a sample interview form.

Interview Questions

There is a wide range of interviewing methods available. Your format of choice may be influenced by the person specification you are trying to match. Irrespective of the technique selected, the interviewers must:

- Ask relevant questions. Know what types of questions are illegal.
- Ensure that all questions are related to selection criteria.
- Keep the interviews consistent.
- Give applicants details of terms and conditions of employment.
- Tell applicants when they can expect to hear about the results of the interview.

Prepare an interview proforma, which is followed, for each person. This should cover the following questions:

1) Find out why the candidate is applying for the job.
2) Ask for examples of the following:
   - How they work
   - Organisational skills
   - Coping with different demands and tasks
   - Working under pressure
   - Working with difficult people
3) Request medical information and, if appropriate, a medical reference.
4) Ask about availability for work.
5) Find out how much they know about the practice, then proceed to fill in the gaps.
6) Ask if they have any questions for you.
7) Finally, ask <u>IF</u> they received a job offer, would they accept?

The Interview Room

Try to avoid confrontational room layouts, such as sitting face to face at a table. Be friendly, use open relaxed body language, and avoid physical barriers. Create comfort with a preliminary chat to establish rapport. When the interview begins, ask if you can take notes. Always give your full attention to the applicant when they are speaking directly to you.

The communication balance should be 80% applicant – 20% interviewer.

The Provisional Job Offer

Be aware that the job offer is the basis of the employment contract. Always state if the offer is subject to satisfactory references. Send out a letter of acceptance for your chosen candidate to sign. Do not officially reject all other candidates until your chosen candidate has accepted the offer – if that person accepts an offer from another company, for example, you might want to reach out to your second choice. That will be awkward if you already sent a courtesy letter dismissing the other candidates.

Appendix 5.1: Interview Record Form

Name of Applicant...
Position Applied For..
Date of Interview..
Interviewer..

SUMMARY OF INTERVIEW

Specifications	Weighting (Mark out of)	Marks Awarded and Why
1.	/5	
2.	/10	
3.	/5	
4.	/10	
5.	/10	
6.	/5	
7.	/10	
8.	/10	
Total score	/65	

COMMENTS

Is this candidate suitable for the position?

When is the candidate available to start work?

Do we want to proceed with this application? – comments

INTERVIEW RESULTS

	Yes / No	**Date**
Shortlisted		
Job offer		
Refusal		
Hold on file		

Signed... Date...............................

Interview Summary:	Satisfactory	Unsatisfactory
Appearance		
Personality		
Relevant experience		
Availability		
Ease of travel		
Enthusiasm		
Overall		

Interviewer's name
Interviewer's signature
Date

Note: An employer must give job applicants the right to see a copy of these notes made about them at interview.

6

Quality Management

Quality in Dental Care

> *Quality* is not a project or a programme. It is never-ending and forever.
> Edwards Deming.

The Receptionists Role for Quality Management

Over recent years, the principles of quality management have been increasingly applied to ensure that health and social care provisions are developed and managed in ways that provide service users with maximum benefits. It's also true to say that when services are designed and delivered based on quality principles, the practice and its employees also reap the benefits.

Theories of quality management and their application have been gaining popularity since the 1930s; quality theorists have introduced and adapted existing techniques for businesses strategies to optimise their effectiveness and efficiency. The Health and Social Care Act 2008 has highlighted the need for understanding of the practical application of high-quality care from being a good asset for the business, to be an essential requirement. There are a wide range of approaches to quality management, applying techniques for assessing and developing aspects of efficiency and effectiveness in the context of Care Quality Commission compliance.

A team approach towards quality management creates a lead role so that senior staff can oversee the practical implementation of policies and procedures. The reception lead role is one example.

Health and Social Care Act 2008

Whole-Team Professionalism

In an ideal world, all dental practices would work to the gold standard in all that they do, from using the best materials and techniques for treating patients to having a fully equipped decontamination room with a wide range of safeguarding policies and protocols

Dental Reception and Supervisory Management, Second Edition. Glenys Bridges.
© 2019 John Wiley & Sons Ltd. Published 2019 by John Wiley & Sons Ltd.
Companion website: www.wiley.com/go/bridges/dental

in place. It is beyond doubt that most practices aim to secure *best practice standards* in all they do. However, some do not, and really, shouldn't be seeing patients at all!

Definitions

Best practice	Methods or techniques that have consistently shown results better those achieved with other means, and are used as benchmarks.
Good practice	Are a set of standards or requirements set by authoritative bodies to achieve the stated objectives.

For some considerable time now, the *idea* of whole-team professionalism has been the way forward for both excellent patient care and career satisfaction for dental care professionals. Over the years, new initiatives such as clinical governance and dental care professional (DCP) registration have been introduced but have only inched us forward with this aspiration.

In some practices, their team ethos, along with the implementation of a wide range of team development initiatives have allowed DCPs to thrive and grow. Without exception, these practices have reaped the benefits of their team's development input. However, such practices are small compared to the greater majority in which very little has changed despite, dental nurse registrations and the requirements it places on registrants.

The Care Quality Commission (CQC) quality initiative is designed to drive quality management in the health and social care sector and provide a robust framework for whole team professionalism. Beginning in April 2010, the CQC required for all providers of health and social care to register and provide evidence of meeting key performance indicators (KPI) for a set of 28 standards outlining the ideal outcome patients should experience when using a service as set out in the CQC's 'Essential Standards of Quality and Safety'. In 2015, these standards were replaced with the Fundamental Standards – Regulated Activities 2014. Plus, a new inspection regime was based on Key Lines of Enquiry (KLOE).

Those practices in which quality principles have been built into their existing activities will find meeting the CQC standards straightforward. When the whole team has involved the workload of CQC compliance, duties are shared, and individuals will own the measures introduced, they will become more productive.

The Role of Policy and Procedure

Policies and procedures are a vital part of business management because they enable managers to make consistent decisions relevant to the business' agreed objectives, set out in the business plan. With this platform in place, employees have standards to measure their performance. A policy manual compiles the organisational policies and standard operating procedures and makes them readily accessible.

Purpose

A policy manual is a systematic, written presentation of company policies, operating procedures, decision-making guidelines, and steps to enforcement. It gives structure and order to a company and its operations.

Development

The management team takes charge of policy and procedure development and guide-lines for enforcement and oversees the creation of the policy manual.

Users

Access to policy manuals on paper or in an electronic format should be provided to new employees as part of their induction. Electronic versions using cloud-based technology are both more accurate and more environmentally friendly. In this format, the team have continuous access to the policies and procedures they are expected to observe.

Continuous Improvement

The most consistent messages running through all new dental regulation is the need for constant improvement and the importance of placing patients' well-being at the core of practice processes. Dental professionals are required to ensure they deliver oral and general health gains in a safe, patient centred environment.

In the past, if a practice appeared orderly and caring, it would have been assumed that the practice was providing good-quality dentistry. However, the days of the public auto-matically trusting professional groups of all kinds are long gone. Today, organisations like the CQC and PCT/LHB will expect to see *proof* that essential standards are set, monitored, standardised, and sustained. Quality management provides a necessary route to the structured and systematic delivery of dental care.

Quality management may be seen as being a considerable organisational and financial burden for the practice owner. They consider that the effort is taken to ensure all the quality management processes are in place eats into their clinical and family time.

However, there is a far more productive way of meeting the demands of quality man-agement. With appropriate training, senior dental nurses are perfectly capable of taking on leadership roles in areas such as decontamination and cross infection control, radia-tion and radiological protection, and care coordination. This training would provide them with knowledge and understanding of quality management principles and pro-cesses along with the technical aspects of each subject area. A well-trained dental nurse would not only be more cost effective but better placed than the dentist to ensure the standards are met in practice.

Regulatory authorities state that the level of this learning should be at least at a super-visory management level (level 3). A level 3 qualification is equivalent to the A-level standard of academic achievement.

Quality Theory

Engineer and statistician Walter Shewhart are widely considered to be the father of modern quality management. During the early 1930s, he introduced the Shewhart learning cycle consisting of four continuous steps; Plan, Do, Study, Act. This concept combines statistical analysis with creative management thinking and is the underlying principle for quality initiatives widely used in dental practices such as clinical govern-ance, CQC standards, and the BDA Good Practice Scheme.

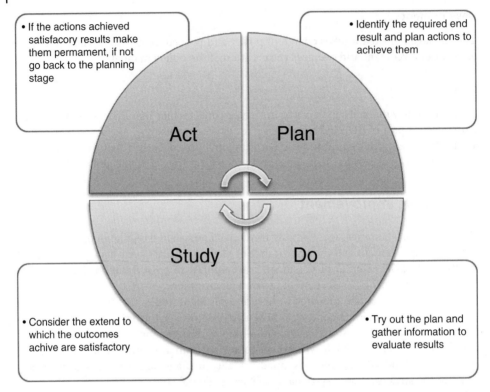

• If the actions achieved satisfacory results make them permament, if not go back to the planning stage

• Identify the required end result and plan actions to achieve them

Act

Plan

Study

Do

• Consider the extend to which the outcomes achive are satisfactory

• Try out the plan and gather information to evaluate results

Figure 6.1 PDSA cycle. *Source:* Van Vliet, V. (2011). *PDCA Cycle.* ToolsHero: https://www.toolshero.com/problem-solving/pdca-cycle-deming.

The quality concept was further developed by one Shewhart's students, W. Edwards Deming, who describes the PDSA spiral (see Figure 6.1):

• **P**lan what to do.
• **D**o it.
• **S**tudy the results.
• **A**ct to make corrections.

The CQC standards are based on the principles of quality management first developed in the United States during the 1930s by Dr. W. Edwards-Deming, an American statistician and consultant, and further established by a wide range of theorists such as Duran and Crosby as the theories of total quality management we work with today. Although the principles began in the United States, they were further developed in the industrialisation of Japan following WWII. The Japanese adaptations of the theory are known as kaizen.

Total quality management (TQM) is a comprehensive and structured approach to organisational management that seeks to improve the quality of products and services through ongoing refinements in response to continuous feedback. TQM processes are divided into the plan, do, check, and act categories (the *PDCA cycle*).

In the *planning* phase, people define the problem to be addressed, collect relevant data, and ascertain the problem's cause. In the *doing* stage, people develop and implement a solution, and decide on a measurement to gauge its effectiveness. In the *checking* aspect, people confirm the results through before-and-after data comparison. In the *acting* phase, people document their findings, inform others about process changes, and make recommendations for the problem to be addressed in the next PDCA cycle.

Kaizen is the Japanese for 'improvement' or 'change for the better' refers to philosophy or practices that focus on continuous improvement of processes supporting business processes, and management. It has been applied in healthcare, psychotherapy, life-coaching, government, banking, and many other industries. When used in the business sense and applied to the workplace, kaizen refers to activities that continually improve all functions, and involves all employees. Kaizen influenced US business and quality management teachers who visited the country and has since spread throughout the world.

There can be no doubt that to observe these detailed standards practices will need the involvement and cooperation of each member. This will make adding the role of treatment coordinator a sensible way to enable practices to allocate responsibility for the development of patient-focused, quality initiatives to ensure that the practice is proactive in observing outcome 1–3 in respect of patient involvement and informed consent.

In recent years, many dental practices have chosen to participate in quality assurance initiatives such as BDA Good Practice and Investors in People and so are familiar with principles of continuous improvement through effective and efficient policies and procedures. For those practices, the quality principles are already built into their activities and taking existing measures forward to meet the CQC standards is straightforward. When the whole team is involved in the development and audit of the standards, not only is the load shared, but individuals are committed to making the measures introduced work. Figure 6.2 illustrates a continuous improvement cycle.

Figure 6.2 Continuous improvement cycle. *Source:* Van Vliet, V. (2011). *PDCA Cycle.* ToolsHero: https://www.toolshero.com/ problem-solving/pdca-cycle-deming.

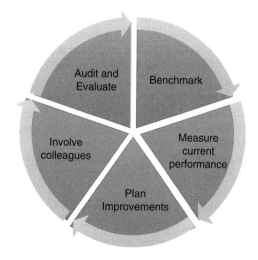

Total Quality Management (TQM)

TQM became a key feature of management during the 1980s. At that time, managers were starting to recognise the value of person-centred approaches to all aspects of their businesses:

TOTAL =	involving everyone in all company activities
QUALITY =	conforming to requirements
MANAGEMENT =	supervision of processes and procedures
TQM =	a process for continuous management of quality

Edwards-Deming's mathematical background had a considerable influence on his thinking and his quality management techniques. He placed great importance on the responsibility of management both at individual and company levels and theorised that 94% of quality problems are the responsibility of management. To address this, he developed a 14-point management philosophy, relevant to organisations of all sizes across all business sectors. These 14 points are now regarded as a recipe for quality, providing guidance and support for managers. They open the mind to systematic ways of thinking about the purpose of the business, its procedures and processes, while considering the roles and needs of its people.

Policy Building

Policies are measures designed to achieve consistent management success, which is the direct result of a clear management direction. In today's business environment, managers need to develop an extensive range of skills to secure an appropriate balance between profitability and compliance with an extensive range of legal and ethical obligations.

Policy writing begins with a statement of purpose and goes on to identify broad guidelines for achieving the stated purpose. As shown in Figure 6.3, this then is a framework for decision-making and defining implementation measures.

Policies should meet identified needs while reflecting the practice's beliefs, values, or philosophies on the issue concerned. The policy will formulate and define simple procedures to be followed to enable a consistent and equitable approach to be adopted. Quality is compromised when no policies are in place, or when policies are vague, badly communicated, or where there is a diversity of interests and preferences, resulting in conflicting objectives amongst those who are directly involved.

Intelligent application of policy is vital; you need discretion in its implementation; however, the margins for that discretion should be stated as part of the policy to prevent it from becoming impotent.

When creating a policy, you should begin with the business plan, which is the managers' constant reference point for decision-making. A comprehensive business plan will identify where the business wants to be in one year and specify how you plan to get there. It will identify targets, budgets, and resources, and then go on to set timetables. With this valuable document in place, the manager has tools to think with.

Having set your goals, a consistent pathway is required to achieve success. At this point, the manager needs agreed policies to move the plan forward. Policy making is

Purpose

- States the outcomes the policy aims to achieve.

Scope

- States who will need to observe to policy.

Relevance

- Lists the regulations Key Lines of Enquiry and guidance that will be met by observing the policy and procedures.

Procedures

- Defines the actions that must be taken to observe the policy.

Audit

- This process establishes the extent to which the policy is fit for purpose; and how improvements can be made.

Review

- Determines how frequently the policy will be audited reviewed.

Figure 6.3 Framework for decision-making and defining implementation measures.

strategic management. Policies are built on the following series of decisions about the area covered by the policy.

Making Improvements

Making improvements to deficient systems can be complicated. This is especially true if improving in one area leads to deterioration in another, or when applying a solution to a problem makes the problem worse. If a system is underperforming, responding with a knee-jerk solution to send the staff on a training course when the real cause of the problem is ineffective procedures, the training course will not fix the problem.

Before making a change, use the quality cycle to understand the bigger picture, wherein problems occur and their domino effects. Discuss your ideas with the team; there are always people who think a change will fail. Find them and ask them why they think this, so you do not find them saying after the event, 'I could have told you why that would fail.'

Systemic Shortfalls

When you address systemic shortfalls, staff motivation often changes in response, and people will then actively seek the knowledge they need to become competent in a new way. A key measure of management success is the quality of care delivered by the practice in both clinical and nonclinical areas of care. Managers need to be aware not only of the operational needs of the practice but must also have a clear vision of the bigger picture and base their management decisions on it, thus ensuring consistency and fairness.

The QUIET quality-focused management process enhances consistent and focused management.

Q	Quality focused: Manager need to have a benchmark for the services they provide and using it as the basis for developing the policies and procedures.
U	Underpinning the work of the team: Leadership and resources are provided to ensure that as far as possible, clinicians can be patient-focused and not distracted by avoidable administrative errors and cumbersome procedures.
I	Information-based management: Management decision needs to be evidence-based, requiring managers to draw information from colleagues and patients when making management decisions.
E	End-user focused: In addition to being evidence-based, discretionary decisions should be holistically based, considering the physical, social, and emotional impacts on purchasers and providers.
T	Team driven: Managers need to motivate and empower the team through good communications and positive strokes.

The role of the reception lead is both pastoral and remedial. This can mean that you are wearing many different hats, at times acting as a matrix band holding different facets of the practice together or serving as a mentor providing support and guidance to colleagues (see Figure 6.4).

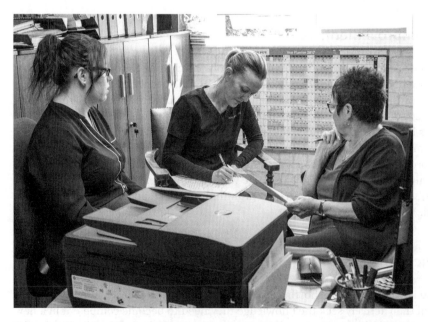

Figure 6.4 The role of the reception lead can mean that you are wearing many different hats.

At other times you will need to *grasp the nettle* to manage complex and often emotionally charged situations. The role of the reception lead is both demanding and rewarding the appropriate skills and support.

It is all too easy for leads to focus on the needs of the patients and colleagues, while failing to recognise their own needs. The fact is, just like the man chopping down trees with a blunt axe, managers that stop to take time for their personal and professional development can reap the benefits and achieve better results for less effort.

Quality Audit

Quality audit is a process for measuring how well systems and procedures do the following:

- Achieve their objectives.
- Use resources.

Edwards-Deming introduced the quality audit approach; it will come as no surprise that his quality audit processes use statistical measures. Deming goes on to state that 'quality systems must be *effective, efficient, and continuously improving*'.

Effectiveness is a measurement on a scale of 1–10 of the extent to which the system secures the desired results (see Figure 6.5). This measure calculates performance to the policy statement, where the objectives for the activity being audited are specified.

Efficiency is again a measure on the scale of 1–10 of the way the system uses resources. The efficiency of a system considers:

- *Economy*. Is the system economical regarding its use of materials and time, and is it cost-effective?
- *Adaptability*. Can the system respond when adapted response is required?
  User friendliness:
  – Are the team trained to operate the system?
  – How does the team experience the system?
  – How do the patients experience the system?
- *Reliability*. Does the system produce consistent results?

Quality audits should be completed regularly to ensure that policies and procedures are fit for purpose and achieved the best results for patients

Theory in Practice

Implementation of quality-audit processes based on the PDCA quality cycle shown in Figure 6.1 starts with the production of benchmarks in the form of a quality statement for the activity. Based on this, an assessment of effectiveness and efficiency from which quality improvements can be determined to raise the overall score achieved when adding together the five individual scores linked to effectiveness and efficiency. It is advisable to involve all users of the system in the process of planning and implementing the improvements which will then be quality audited.

Effectiveness	Score out of 10	Analysis
	3	There is often a lack of clarity about who is responsible for decontamination activities. At times there too many nurses in the decontamination room, at other times nobody is available, and we run out of stock and available instruments. There have been numerous incidents of instruments going missing.

Efficiency	Score out of 10	Analysis
Economy	3	Patients have been reappointed due to lack if usable instruments and at times we have needed to obtain materials quickly, rather than economically. This is due in part to the fact that there are only 2 autoclaves and 1 washer-disinfector for 8 surgeries. One of the sterilizers is unreliable we can't always spare the time to use the t use the washer disinfector. There are only 2 ultrasonic baths are regularly overloaded with instruments.
Reliability	3	The lack of resources: equipment, staff and time mean that our decontamination processes are often deficient.
Adaptability	3	The general lack of resources and organisation mean that we are frequently unable to respond to unexpected events and the service to patients suffers as a direct result.
User Friendly	1	In no way can this be user friendly unless things are changed. The quality control of the processing of instruments is dubious.

Figure 6.5 Effectiveness and efficiency analysis. *Source:* Business Dictionary, Quality circles. http://www.businessdictionary.com/definition/quality-circle-QC.html.

Policy, Process, and Procedure

At a strategic level, quality management is the development of a quality policy defining benchmarks, objectives, procedures, and processes. A quality policy is an *umbrella policy* covering a range of subpolicies, each related to specific areas of activity. Together, they define the operational aspect of quality management, starting with the strategic policy statement, in the form of a general statement of intent, outlining the practice philosophy, ethics, and goals. For example:

- Continuous improvement
- Company and employee attitudes
- Achieve customer satisfaction
- Identify needs

- Involve everyone
- Set service standards
- Measure results
- Continuous professional development
- Recognise and reward

   With a clear view of what you are working to achieve in respect of quality management, you are now ready to identify the procedures that will secure success. Consider how you will:

- Motivate staff
- Produce clear work instructions
- Conduct quality audit procedures
- Monitor procedures
- Market research effects
- Recognise staff achievements

Quality Circles in Practice

It is increasingly clear that quality management is at its best when the whole team is engaged and understands how their role contributes to the overall quality of patient care; and most importantly, to the 'patient experience' at your practice.

Spreading the Workload of Quality Creation

With the best will in the world, without the support of their teams, registered managers and providers cannot create a workplace environment in which the quality of care is continuously improving. In most professional healthcare practices, the registered provider is actively engaged in fee-earning activities, which make it difficult to keep a watchful eye on the work of each team member. Their main priority is quite rightly the patient in your chair. The only way to consistently achieve continuously improving, high-quality, well-led care is to ensure that each member is as dedicated to the provision of care excellence, as are their leaders and managers.

Quality Circles Create an Inclusive, Whole-Team Environment

The enduring principle of quality management is the creation of working practices that are effective, efficient, and continuously improving. Such systems do not develop by luck; they require focused efforts from everyone in the team. Management can direct such efforts by communicating what needs to be done in practice policy, specifying the most efficient ways to secure the desired results in related procedures. This process does not end when the policies and procedures are in place at this point the Continuously Improving aspect of quality management kicks-in based on the experiences of the system's users, a quality circle provides channels for the team to feedback and input new ideas.

Team Perspectives Can Shape Quality Improvements

The users of quality management systems include the practice team, who have unique up-close and personal insight of the quality of your practice's services. This insight is the cornerstone of quality development. When given an outlet and receiving a solution-focused mindset using techniques such as significant event analysis, the DCP can experience reflective learning at its best through analysis of both the team's triumphs and incidents of underperformance.

Create Productive Team Relationships

Effective, respectful communication between all parts of the practice is essential for quality development. When DCPs consider the management as being distant and remote, it is unlikely that there will be mutual respect, and it is even less likely that different parts of the practice team will understand or care about the challenges and frustrations of their colleagues. A quality circle provides chances for all team members to share their experiences.

Quality Summary

The system in Figure 6.5 has scored 13 out of a possible 50. This reflects a 26% quality rating. Were the CQC to visit, they would be far from happy. On the surface, the decontamination room looks well equipped with sterilisers, ultrasonic baths, and steriliser pouches, etc., but if someone were to observe how the resources are being used, they might pick up on the points shown in the analysis above.

Based on these observations, a team meeting is required to discuss an action plan to rectify these shortfalls and raise the quality rating to at least 80% in the first instant, and then based on continuous improvement on to 95–100%.

7

Working as a Team

To work well as a team requires the individual team members to have a range of skills and aptitudes. By far, the most important of these are communication skills. This chapter looks at the interpersonal skills identified by Daniel Goleman in his book *Working with Emotional Intelligence*. When working as a team, we depend on our colleagues having the work-based competencies required to enable them to play their role effectively; this links to their IQ. People are a pleasure to work with when they have the type of communication skills, connected to emotional intelligence (EQ).

The colleagues with whom we enjoy working and with whom we produce our best work are those with whom we form bonds of trust and understanding. Most people have a fundamental need to connect with the people they spend their working day with and can feel unsettled when for any reason they are unable to communicate comfortably with them. In some cases, this happens when a supervisor with a high quota of EQ joins a dysfunctional team and introduces a new range of interpersonal skills, with hopes of transforming the team.

For some years now, educationalists have expressed their concerns about the effects of children spending an excessive number of hours in front of the television or on electronic devices such as iPads or smart phones, noting these children do not learn how to interact with others. Their research has shown that 4 out of 10 such children are unable to co-work, more than half of them lack the motivation to perform tasks, such as homework, and their listening and oral skills are deficient. All of this is detrimental to their ability to integrate into a work team.

Now that continuous personal professional development is an integral part of dental professionalism, teams need to invest time and energy in the development of skills that enable them to understand each other's needs and communicate their own needs, so that they can create a working environment in which they can flourish. This starts with the development of personal competencies, including self-awareness and self-management, and social awareness; in this way, they become able to recognise the needs and feelings of others and so are better able to manage workplace relationships.

The Role of Management and Leadership

In this section, we will examine ways management and leadership skills can be used to build trusting, respectful relationships.

Dental Reception and Supervisory Management, Second Edition. Glenys Bridges.
© 2019 John Wiley & Sons Ltd. Published 2019 by John Wiley & Sons Ltd.
Companion website: www.wiley.com/go/bridges/dental

> **Management** is concerned with ensuring services and procedures run to plan and deliver on promises.
> **Leadership** is concerned with developing services and procedures to inspire and support people.

For managers and leaders, it is a significant advantage to be able to tune into the needs and expectations of others. To do this requires the skill of empathy. Several highly intelligent people lack this skill, whereas other people who are considered not to have a high IQ can often possess real insight into their own and other people's needs. These people are deemed to have a high EQ.

Leaders and managers with high EQs effortlessly create person-focused teams, because this is how they naturally relate to others. Wise bosses will recognise the value of innate qualities such as empathy, organisational awareness, and service. They seek out people with these qualities to ensure the whole team benefits from their inclusion.

Empathy	• a sense of the emotions and views of others
Organisational awareness	• responsiveness to team politics and culture
Service	• the desire to identify and meet the needs of clients and colleagues

Nature and Nurture

Not everyone can develop EQ, so when recruiting, identify applicants' attitudes, values, and beliefs, as they reveal an individual's EQ:

- *Beliefs* are the most superficial level of interpretation. We form our beliefs through casual observation and use them to evaluate people and situations. Beliefs are, however, easily changed when new information shows the belief to be incorrect. For example, if you think that it is raining outside, you may consider someone is going out without an umbrella to be foolish. If you then discover that the rain has stopped, you would revise your opinion on that behaviour.
- *Attitudes* are deeper seated. They arise from our family and cultural background. To change an attitude is more complex than changing a belief. It involves social pressure and development. Over recent years social attitudes towards smoking in public, drinking and driving, and working mothers have shifted considerably.
- *Values* are central to our personalities; they make us the people we are and are the single-most influential tool of interpretation.

Team Roles and Related Behaviours

The beauty of working in a team is that each person can contribute what he or she does best, and with the help of colleagues develop areas of weakness. This aspect of teamwork should be managed by the lead so that the business benefits rather than suffers from the diversity in the team. The ideal team consists of individuals whose roles complement each other and so add strength to the team. The strengths and aptitudes of individuals is an important consideration when appointing tasks between team members and also for staff selection. For example, if recruiting a receptionist, do not choose someone who wants to take a nursing role. Team roles must be clearly defined and match the needs and personality both of the business and the individual.

In 1965, Dr. Bruce Tuckman proposed four stages of group development, forming, storming, norming, and performing (a fifth stage, adjourning, was later added). A British research and management theorist, Dr. Raymond Meredith Belbin, studied numerous teams and identified links between personality traits and success in work roles. His nine team roles described how team members can contribute and interact while they work through these stages.[1]

When the employer can match the personality to the work role, the chances of maintaining a viable team are increased. The quality of teamwork and team spirit are closely linked. In-group situation individuals are influenced to behave in specific ways. The influences that cause us to act are primarily centred in our value systems. People cannot be comfortable when forced to take action that does not support their values.

We each have a preferred role in any group. As shown in Figure 7.1, some people are natural leaders and others will look to them for leadership. Others are reflectors or questioners. Before some individuals can become a part of a dynamic group, they must travel through Tuckman's stages of team formation. Belbin said that team roles affect how that is accomplished. The characteristics of four of Belbin's team roles most appropriate to dental teams are discussed next. Consider the task each member of your team is most suited to and identify their contribution to the team.

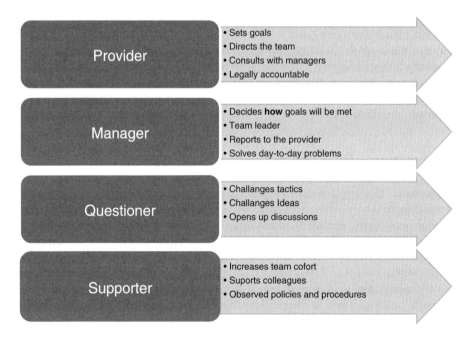

Figure 7.1 Preferred roles. Adapted from Belbin's team roles.

---

1 https://www.belbin.com/resources/blogs/belbin-and-tuckman

Stage 1 FORMING

The initial stage that groups of individuals pass through on route to becoming a functioning team. New groups initially need to test their leadership. At this stage, individuals looked to the leader for direction, and based on the quality of leadership will decide whether to join the group. Initially, conversations will be on safety issues. However, gradually grumbling about the setting will occur and this will lead on to the storming stage.

Stage 2 STORMING

At this stage, the group members are vying for their positions in the group. Here, the following behaviour occurs dependant on people's preferred defence mechanisms. Some people will become defensive and decide not to join the fray; they will stand back and allow others to compete. Other people will form cliques to isolate anyone that the clique does not endorse. Rule breaking will occur.

Stage 3 NORMING

Once the pecking order is established, the group will become motivated; more favourable alliances are formed during storming. Members of the group begin to regard themselves as a group, and harmony increases.

Stage 4 PERFORMING

At this stage, the group increases productiveness, interpersonal issues are settled, and there is a strong drive towards goals.

At times, the group will backslide, and the comfort of stage 4 returns to the conflict of stages 2 and 3. This can happen when a new member joins the team or at times of other significant changes. It is vital that the manager is sensitive to the dynamics of the team at all times and acts to strengthen and support as required, in line with practice policy and the needs of individuals.

Communication – The Cement of Society

All of the most successful teams have something in common; they are excellent communicators.

Your chances of being successful at anything you increase if you can communicate well. In most cases, when people communicate well and make their needs, thoughts, or feeling understood others would take them more seriously and make more effort to co-operate with them.

When people become exasperated, they will adopt less cooperative ways of behaving, using childish behaviour that has worked for them in the past, which may well be difficult to deal with.

Some people are better than others at dealing with difficult people; they seem to have been born with natural energy and confidence. Others must work to develop the personal skills that help us to communicate well when others are not. In this section of the course, we will look at communication skills.

Defence Mechanisms

Ideally, we all want to feel satisfied, safe and happy. Our actions are intended to create this state. When we feel dissatisfied, unsafe, or unhappy and not able to rectify this with co-operative communication, then we resort to defending ourselves using our preferred defence mechanisms. For some, this means activating their fight instincts; meaning they become aggressive and argumentative, whereas others prefer to adopt a fight instinct and avoid the issue or overlook the matters at hand. Either way, these are difficult responses for supervisors to handle unless they can understand the motives behind the behaviour.

Burnout

Researchers have shown that people who work with people are most likely to suffer from 'burnout' when the stress of dealing with people becomes too much. Burnout is the term used when you lose interest and motivation and begin to think negatively. Burnout happens when you have been under intense stress for some time, or when you have been giving others too much emotional support for a long time.

Working Successfully with Difficult People

Risk Factors

Factors that place workers at risk of violence in the workplace include interacting with the public, exchanging money, delivering services or goods, working late at night or during early morning hours, working alone, guarding valuable assets, or property, and dealing with aggressive people in volatile situations.

Prevention

Practice policies and strategies have the potential for reducing the risk of workplace violence. The table in Figure 7.2 lists practical ways to prevent aggression both from the public and also within the team Examples of prevention strategies include systems for:

- Initial responses
- Post-incident analysis
- Action planning to prevent recurrences

No single strategy is appropriate for all workplaces, but all workers and employers should assess the risk of violence in their workplaces and take appropriate action to reduce those risks (see Chapter 8). A workplace violence prevention programme should include a system for:

- Documenting incidents
- Procedures in the event of incidents
- Open communication between employers and workers

Preventing aggression from Patients	Preventing aggression within the team
Visibility - Good lighting throughout price premises	Clear work allocation
Cash-handling policies	Working produces and protocols
Physical separation of workers and customers	Detailed inductions
Security devices, e.g. CCTV	Appoint mentors
Effective complaints handling	Open-door approach to problems
Staff to give an excellent service	Manage personality clashes

Figure 7.2 Practical ways to prevent aggression from the public and within the team.

Problem Recognition and Empathy

People's behaviour becomes challenging when they have a need that they do not feel has been satisfied. Your first thought must be to identify which particular frustration is causing the problem at hand and then to concentrate on problem-solving. To manage your people in such situations, you need to find out what they perceive as being the cause of their lack of satisfaction. In most cases, one of the following four categories will apply. They feel that:

- You don't care about them.
- You have broken your promises.
- You are incompetent.
- No one listens to them.

Once the causes are identified, it will become clearer how to respond effectively.

Managing Angry People

Patients and colleagues may become angry when they have a need that has not been met and they believe that *you* should have satisfied that need (see Figure 7.3). At such times, it is more useful to focus on the feelings rather than the problem.

Use empathy – put yourself in their shoes. Say things such as:

I can see why you are not happy; I would feel the same if this happened to me.

Follow these steps:

1) Listen carefully to what they have to say and give feedback on what you understand from what they are saying.
2) Then deal with the problem. If you cannot do what the person wants, you need to, offer alternatives. Don't stress what you *cannot* do; instead, plan what you *could* do.
3) Be solution-focused rather than problem-focused.

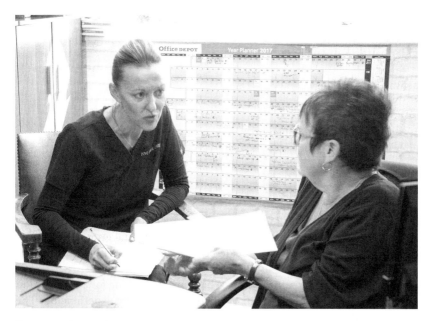

Figure 7.3 Aggressive team interactions.

Handling Aggressive Incidents

- Use assertive nonverbal language.
- Encourage the potential aggressor to talk.
- Give reassurance that you are working for a win-win outcome.
- Proceed gradually. Anticipate violence.
- Do not leave yourself open and vulnerable.
- Avoid audiences, but do not isolate yourself from the aggressor.

Working with an Aggressor

- Break the issue down into parts.
- Offer alternatives.
- Structure the aggressor's expectations.
- Present both sides of the argument.
- Use facts.
- Request for delayed compliance.
- Avoid making the aggressor lose face.
- Use praise freely.

Post-Incident Helping

The person needs understanding, comfort and warmth, and to:

- Understand what happened.
- Adjust to it.

- Talk about the incident.
- Overcome the feelings of loss of control and self-blame.
- Regain regular patterns of behaviour.
- Relax.
- Explore the way forward.

Learn the lessons and move on. *The practice needs to:*

- Make an accurate record of the incident, agreed by any witnesses present.
- Review policy and protocol.

Workplace Bullying

When I write about bullying in dental teams, I always receive calls from dental care professionals being bullied at work. Bullying is widespread in dental groups, and when I found myself on the receiving end of it, I decided to study social psychology, to understand what was happening and why.

Many readers attracted to articles on workplace bullying are looking for a magic wand to wave over their problems to relieve them of the distress they are experiencing. The article might define bullying and outline coping strategies.

Bullying is not an exclusively downward phenomenon; I have met as many practice managers and dental employers being bullied by subordinates as employees being bullied by managers or employers.

It is a mistake to jump too quickly to the conclusion that you are a helpless victim of workplace bullying; you are well advised to consider other explanations for interpersonal problems you may be experiencing. In some cases, the real problem is a mismatch between personalities. Another person interacting with the 'bully' may not have any problem with them.

Bullying can take many forms; in dental teams, it often includes one or more of the following:

- Constant fault-finding – the triviality, regularity, and frequency betray bullying. There is usually a grain of truth (but only a grain) in the criticism, leading you to believe the criticism is valid, which it may well not be.
- Simultaneous with the criticism is a constant refusal to acknowledge your achievements.
- Continually attempting to undermine your status.
- When in a workgroup, being singled out and treated differently; for instance, everyone else can get away with murder but the moment you put a foot wrong – however trivial – action is taken against you.
- Being isolated excluded from what's going on.
- Being belittled demeaned and patronised, especially in front of others.
- Having your responsibilities increased, but your authority is taken away.
- Imposing on you unrealistic goals or deadlines set, which change as you approach them.
- Finding what you have said is twisted, distorted, and misrepresented.
- Being subjected to disciplinary procedures with verbal or written warnings imposed for trivial or fabricated reasons and without proper investigation.

What Can You Do?

When we have formed a view about people, we see only what best fits our version of them. This gives rise to 'scapegoat' mentality, which I find to be commonplace in dental teams. As individuals, we have cultural beliefs about acceptable and unacceptable qualities in others. These judgments result from our educational and social status. As dental teams draw from a full span of social and educational groups, it is not surprising that problems occur so frequently.

Don't let problems pile up. Take responsibility for your role in events. If you have been too submissive and allowed yourself to be dominated, you need to recognise this and consider finding positive ways to respond to the bullies; your newfound assertiveness could gain their respect.

Bullies may make you feel ashamed, embarrassed, guilty, or afraid – this is understandable, but you must challenge these feelings, talking them through with someone you respect and trust. These feelings provide bullies with their power base for controlling and silencing their victims. Talk to someone; you cannot handle bullying by yourself.

Communicate with Care

You may have an exceptionally caring attitude towards those around you, but it will count for very little unless you know how to put it across. Communicating with care is letting others know that what they think and feel is of concern to you.

Here are five golden rules of excellent communication in your working relationships:

1) *Be sincere.* This is the foundation of a good relationship. You cannot relate well to others if you present a false face. Sincerity encourages trust.
2) *Be positive about others.* Look for the positives in those around you. Tell them what you like about them.
3) *Be clear and assertive.* Present a confident, positive outlook that springs from self-worth.
4) *Be appropriate.* Take time to understand the other person. Look at things from their viewpoint and consider their age and background.
5) *Be interested.* Always listen to people and learn about them. To show that you are curious, you should:

   - Give them feedback.
   - Do not dominate the conversation.
   - Use body language.
   - Look for nonverbal cues.

8

Team Meetings

Introduction

Team meetings are essential for effective team communications. In busy workplaces it's a mistake to expect people to maintain productive relationships unless at some point they can receive information from management related to their progress, air their views, and explore new ways to work together as a team.

Team Meetings are not meant to replace the regular essential day-to-day communications between the team leaders and the team; daily discussions should run alongside team meeting procedures. Many practices think that email and mobile phone communications can solve all their communications problems, but they cannot. Team Meeting works because of their face-to-face format, which is essential for all sensitive communications.

Team meetings have several purposes:

- Enable and improve downward, upward, and sideways communications.
- Prevent *rumour mills* and the *grapevine* from gaining credibility.
- Enable clarity of direction and information from the top.
- Enable questions and suggestions to be fed back from all staff to the top.
- Develop greater awareness and involvement at all levels.
- Avert *mushroom management* (keeping people in the dark and covering them with manure).
- Create a culture of open communication.
- Clear blockages and misunderstandings.
- Explain financial, commercial and strategic issues.
- Develop a shared sense of mission, vision, collective aims, and the reasons why.
- Cease reliance or dependence on assumptions.

Structuring Team Meetings

The process for structuring a team meeting has a seven-staged approach:

Dental Reception and Supervisory Management, Second Edition. Glenys Bridges.
© 2019 John Wiley & Sons Ltd. Published 2019 by John Wiley & Sons Ltd.
Companion website: www.wiley.com/go/bridges/dental

Stage 1: Initiation

This is a trigger setting a course of events into motion. Proactive management initiatives are triggered when team leaders consider the best use of resources to achieve the practice's strategic objectives.

Stage 2: Research

Research is a systematic investigation of the facts, conducted before acting to ensure that you don't blunder in blindly. At this point, you assess the resources available and begin to visualise the result, as advocated by Steven Covey in his book *The Seven Habits of Highly Effective People*, in which he advises Team Leaders to 'begin with the end in mind' using a process of questioning followed by due consideration of the information collected. The supervisor increases their understanding of *what* is required and *how* to achieve the necessary results. At this point, you should consider the time and the place to hold the meeting session, and the resources available.

Stage 3: Design

In this stage, the project's framework (*what* needs to be done) is identified. At the design stage, the manager creates the strategy, preparing the way for the planning stage when the practicalities of *how* to proceed are made. The design needs to be detailed and specific. The phrase 'To be terrific, you must be specific' highlights the importance of SMART objectives, as shown in Figure 8.1, that can be audited and evaluated at the appropriate time.

Stage 4: Planning

Planning is the act of formulating a programme for a definite course of action. At this stage, you agree on the practical steps needed to achieve the result and allocate resources. With the practicalities agreed, the initiative progresses.

Using SMART objectives for planning team meetings

SMART Objectives

SMART	Actions
Specific	Set objectives.
Measurable	Determines details such as how much, when, and who.
Achievable	Here you need to consider if the specific and measurable aspects are realistic and can be achieved.
Relevant	Identify how the above contribute to the achievement of the specific objectives.
Time measured	Time the project; define when results are audited and evaluated.

Figure 8.1 Using SMART objectives for planning team meetings.

Stage 5: Implementation

Here the plan is put into action. It is essential to keep a record of events for analysis, noting all aspects where expectations were either exceeded or unattained. Recording this for later analysis enables the definition of best practice for future activities.

Stage 6: Audit

An audit is a project review and examination of facts and figures to assess the results. The audit takes place when the *time measured* aspects of the SMART objectives have elapsed.

Stage 7: Evaluation

In this context, the evaluation essentially looks at whether a programme works. It uses the audits of the facts and figures, plus the thoughts and feelings of those affected by the initiative, to assess the value of the results, compared to the outcomes identified at the design stage of the process.

The planning process is a structured, logical, and methodical management technique enabling supervisors to take a considered approach towards management initiatives. The method uses a staged approach, breaking down the activities at each stage to lead into each other, leaving an audit trail for a final assessment of the success and value of the project.

Communication Aids for a Team Meeting

The Physical Environment

Team briefs are a flexible and effective method for change management, team building, and problem-solving. You can choose any format for your meeting – your options are as broad as your imagination, and you are certainly not limited to off-the-shelf or tried-and-tested formats.

Split big groups into small task groups – this is more dynamic and produces more ideas and gets the whole group working better, particularly when they present ideas and review with the entire group. As with teambuilding exercises, if you split into subteams of more than four, it is advisable to have each team appoint a leader to prevent things from becoming chaotic, with some members becoming 'passengers'.

Facilitating useful team briefs is a skill that comes with experience. There are some important guidelines you need to consider when choosing where to run your team meetings. Make sure you have:

- Enough space for comfort
- A quiet environment to enable effective conversation
- Excellent sight lines for visual aids
- Planned processes/areas to prevent interruptions

Visual Information

To ensure that the meetings participants fully acknowledge and consider the information presented during the meeting, initially provide information verbally, and then backed-up in a visual format. This might take the form of reports, diagrams, graphs, and charts are all of which are valuable tools to reinforce information.

If you have the use of PowerPoint technology the use of attractive slides enables the team to observe and discuss visual information, confirming their recognition and understanding.

Experiential Learning

People learn continually as individuals and as work groups from daily experiences. The term for this type of learning is *experiential learning.* American educational theorist David Kolb said, 'Learning is the process whereby knowledge is created through the transformation of experience'; experiential learning begins with *experience.*[1]

The cycle begins with experiences. In your practice, an example might be when the team leader needs to choose between two actions:

1) We begin by *reflecting* to **identify** the strengths and weaknesses of each option, perhaps asking, 'What does this involve?'
2) Then we **consider** the options to interpret *meaning.*
3) We then **continue to consider** the potential outcomes; make a choice and begin to *plan*
4) Once the plans are in hand, we identify ways to involve others to implement projects (*joint planning*).
5) Then to progress the selected option take the first steps towards *coordinated action.*

Understanding how people learn is the first step towards the selection of the most appropriate learning materials. You will need to have a wide range of materials to hand.

Barriers to Communication

People are often hit with a lot of information in a meeting. The amount that can be taken in and remembered at any one time is limited. That information can be retrieved later, so it needs to be stored appropriately. The *longer a message*, the higher is the chance that information in the middle section will not be properly stored so that it can be correctly retrieved when required.

When we *take things for granted,* it can affect the energy that we spend on registering information. If a *message becomes too familiar,* we can tune it out and thus not pick up on any changes or adaptations, even if they are vital.

People do *need to tune in to* what is being said. When someone gives you information that you were not expecting, it takes a second or two to assimilate that information.

---

1 Kolb, David A. (1984). Experiential Learning: Experience as the Source of Learning and Development. Englewood Cliffs, NJ: Prentice-Hall, Inc., p. 38.

If the presenter does not allow you that time, it can take a while before you can entirely register what is being said.

How the listener feels about the presenter will influence the way we pick up on any message. If the team leader has not established credibility with the team, the leader is less likely to be taken seriously, and less likely to secure the full cooperation of team members. This would also apply if the receivers distrusted the sender for any reason.

Fear is a barrier to retention. Have you ever tried to read a magazine when you have been waiting at the dentist, or for any other important appointment? Remember taking your driving test? Fear releases chemicals into the brain, which alters thinking and concentration.

Structure Information to Assist Remembering

Communication is vital in team meetings. Effective presentation skills will help you to achieve the required outcome. You will also need to show understanding of how you can strengthen verbal communication and manage potential barriers. You will be required to structure the information in this chapter so that you can make a brief presentation to your tutor, who will mark this using the preset criteria included in this handbook. These marks will count towards your final grade.

During your everyday work as a team leader, you will frequently need to communicate information to others verbally. The level of skill that you apply to this process will affect the level of success you achieve. One of the primary activities of management is communication. Verbal communication is vital and should always be constructed in a way that recognises the importance of the communication chain. The process of planning and organising information was illustrated along with the contribution of the listener to the overall success of the communication process.

You may be thinking that presentation skills are not relevant to you in your everyday work. Well, think again, and consider how often you need to communicate verbally to people in your workplace. Consider the value of talking in a logical and considered fashion, whether you are explaining treatment options to a patient or explaining to your employer why it would be beneficial to employ another member of staff. Please list the people with whom you communicate verbally on a day-to-day basis: Each communication is a presentation of a type and should be constructed with thought and consideration for the receiver.

Unless the receiver registers a presentation, it cannot be interpreted. Because each of us is different, we will each place a different interpretation on the same things. This can affect what others remember and understand from what you say. For example, I might say, 'That book was horrific,' meaning that I did not enjoy reading it, whereas someone else could use the same terms as a high recommendation. When making any presentation, we need to, as far as possible, keep the view and likely interpretations of the listener in mind.

A key feature of verbal communication is that the receiver needs to be able to remember the information communicated; otherwise, the value of the discussion is lost. Over recent years psychologists have carried out numerous studies into how we remember information. Although there are many schools of thought cornering the cognitive processes of memory, the fact remains that memory is dependent on three different but related methods: input of information (*registration*), storage (*retention*), and at the appropriate time, retrieval (*remembering*).

Registration

When passing on information to others, it is important to present the information in a way that will assist the other person to understand and retain what has been said. Their previous knowledge and experience are essential to the way in which messages are registered, interpreted, and retrieved. Whenever you need to pass on information, observation and application of the two following theories will help ensure that others remember the information.

Retention

Primary and Recency

One theory of retention is primacy and recency, which advocates that when communicating information, the probability of that information being retained is influenced by where that information is placed in the presentation. The most significant chance of retention lies with the information presented at the beginning of a presentation (primacy) and the end of a presentation (recency).

All good presenters put the theory to use with the standard technique of introducing their presentation with an overview of what they are about to say – the introduction. They then go on to cover the content of the presentation – the material – and then conclude with a brief review – the summary. In this way, the most vital information is reinforced with both primacy and recency.

Spaced Repetition

This theory suggests that the more often we hear a message, the higher the likelihood of retention. If the most vital information of your talk is outlined in the introduction, described in the body of the discussion and then recapped in summary, you will find that the message is more likely to be registered, be remembered, and be retrievable.

Remembering

Remembering, or retrieval of information, can be hindered by several factors. The following are barriers to remembering:

- *Surroundings*. Have you ever tried to carry out a conversation over loud music? A ringing telephone or side conversations will have the same effect.
- *Anxiety*. If the listener is made anxious by their surroundings, it will also limit their attention span and prevent information from registering.
- *Boredom*. If the listener is bored, or just not interested in what you have to say, then the chances of retention are reduced.
- *Distractions*. The same applies if the listener has other things on their mind or if they are being distracted by other events, such as a misbehaving child.

Answering Questions

Your meeting does not end once you have had your say. The question period is often is the part of the meeting that influences the team the most. After all, you have had time to practice the rest of the talk. This is the part of the presentation where your ability to interact with the team will come to the fore. Since you cannot always predict what you will be asked, here are a few guidelines for taking team questions:

1) Always repeat each question, so the entire team knows what you have been asked.
2) Before you answer, take a moment to reflect on the question. By not rushing to respond, you show a degree of respect for the questioner, and you give yourself time to be sure you are answering the question that was asked. If you are unsure, restate the question or ask for a clarification.
3) Above all, wait for the questioner to finish asking the question before you begin your answer! The only exception is when it becomes necessary to break in on a vague, rambling question; this is your show, and you have only a limited time to make your presentation. It is essential, however, that you break in tactfully. Say something like 'So, are you asking....?' This will focus on the question and give you a place to begin an answer. Remember that your ability to interact with a team is also being evaluated.
4) If a question is asked during the talk, and it will clarify an ambiguity, answer it immediately.
5) Postpone questions aimed at resolving specific problems (or arcane knowledge) until the end of the talk or private discussion; this is particularly important if the answer will distract either you or the team away from the flow of your presentation.
6) Avoid prolonged discussions with one person, extended answers, and especially arguments.
7) If you cannot answer a question, say so. Do not apologize. You then may:
   ➤ Offer to research an answer, and then get back to the questioner later.
   ➤ Suggest resources that would help the questioners to address the question themselves.
   ➤ Ask for suggestions from the team.
8) Finish your answer by asking the person who asked that question whether you answered the question sufficiently. This acknowledges and thanks the questioner, it lets the rest of the team feel comfortable asking questions (because it shows you are genuinely interested in addressing team issues, not just in lecturing to them), and it gives you a chance to more fully answer the question if your first effort was not entirely on target.

Gathering Feedback

Feedback gathering enables you to recognise what has worked and could be improved in future meetings. It should be routine for a copy of the feedback from for each session to be collected. Headings for a formal feedback form would gather feedback about:

- The time at which the meeting was held
- The length of the session
- How information was presented

- Whether the meeting answered all questions
- How the format could be improved for future meetings

As with all the team meeting documentation, design materials that will work for your team. *The best ways to do that involve your people by asking for their feedback.*

Team meetings can be very productive when the lead is skilled and aware of the needs of their team. To achieve maximum benefits, try to involve all staff at suitable stages in the planning and presentation stages of the meeting. The process must be seen by your people to be their own – designed with their issues and their practicalities in mind, as well as the communications needs of the practice.

9

Safety and Well Being

Safeguarding

This chapter looks at regulatory requirements in respect of safeguarding children and vulnerable adults. The content will determine practical strategies for receptionists to observe practice policies and protocols, leading to a productive and consistent approach to significant events. The chapter will address issues such as who needs to be involved, how to ensure measures are followed through, and how decisions are made.

Safeguarding Children and Vulnerable Adults

Each member of the dental team has safeguarding responsibilities, both as a health care professional and as members of society. When any of us hear something about a child or vulnerable adult that concerns us, we should report our concerns to someone who can help.

Vulnerable Adults

The term *vulnerable adults* covers an extensive range of individuals, some of whom may be incapable of looking after any aspect of their lives and others who may be experiencing short periods of illness or disability with an associated reduction in their ability to make decisions.[1]

A Stepped Approach to Safeguarding

Safeguarding vulnerable adults is a complex area of practice involving a wide range of services and service providers. It may be difficult at times to identify those with the responsibility to act. Another consideration is whether the adult has decision-making

---

1 British Medical Association (October 2011). *Safeguarding Vulnerable Adults - A Toolkit for General Practitioners.* safeguardingvulnerableadults.pdf.

Dental Reception and Supervisory Management, Second Edition. Glenys Bridges.
© 2019 John Wiley & Sons Ltd. Published 2019 by John Wiley & Sons Ltd.
Companion website: www.wiley.com/go/bridges/dental

capacity or whether decisions need to be made on their behalf. Therefore, this six-step process is recommended:

Step one	Prevention – identifying adults who may be vulnerable
Step two	Assessing the individual's needs
Step three	Responding to harm or abuse – assessing competence
Step four	Responding to harm or abuse – identifying relevant services
Step five	Responding to harm or abuse – taking a consensual approach
Step six	Safeguarding

Principles of Safeguarding Vulnerable Adults

The Department of Health has developed a list of critical principles to determine good practice in for safeguarding vulnerable adults. These are given below and are reflected throughout the following guidance.

Principle 1: Empowerment

These principles presume that adults should oversee their care and of any decisions that affect their lives. Safeguarding must involve promoting the independence and quality of life of adults and must maximise their ability to control their own lives. Where adults cannot make decisions, as a result, e.g. of a lack of capacity to make the specified decision, they should still be involved in the decision as far as possible. Legally and ethically, however, adults with ability have the right to make decisions about their care and treatment, even where those decisions may not be thought to be in their best interests.

Principle 2: Protection

Patients should be offered the support necessary for them to protect themselves. Where adults are less able to protect or promote their interests, health professionals should take reasonable and appropriate measures to ensure their protection by assessing where proactive steps are required to protect people.

Principle 3: Prevention

Prevention of harm or abuse is the primary goal. Prevention involves working with individuals to reduce risks of harm or abuse that they find unacceptable. Prevention involves delivering high-quality person-centred services in safe environments. All adults have a right to holistic care that is focused on their individual needs, including their need to be kept safe.

Principle 4: Proportionality

In addition to respecting the informed choices of competent adults, safeguarding responses should be proportional to the nature and seriousness of the concern. Options should be presented that are the least restrictive of individual rights and choices while remaining a practical treatment option.

Principle 5: Partnership

Safeguarding adults are most useful where individuals, professionals, and communities work together to prevent, detect, and respond to harm and abuse.

Principle 6: Transparency and Accountability

As with all other areas of healthcare delivery, responsibilities for safeguarding should form part of the ongoing assessment and clinical audit to identify areas of concern and to improve care. Proper safeguarding requires collaboration and transparency with partner agencies.

Children

Members of the dental team are not responsible for making a diagnosis of child abuse or neglect, just for sharing concerns appropriately.[2]

Concerns Regarding Abuse

Abuse or neglect may present to the dental team in several different ways: through a direct allegation (sometimes termed a *disclosure*) made by the child, a parent, or some other person through signs and symptoms that are suggestive of physical abuse or neglect or through observations of child behaviour or parent–child interaction.

Because of the frequency of injuries to areas routinely examined during a dental check-up, the dentist has an essential role in intervening on behalf of an abused child. It is assumed that the dentist will be observing a child who is fully dressed. In some instances, the diagnosis of child abuse is evident. However, there are occasions when evidence is inconclusive, and the diagnosis merely suspected. If in doubt, you should always take advice from Children's Social Services.

When a situation arises, it is vital that the team has a planned process in place. Please see the flowchart in Figure 9.1.

Referrals

It is best practice to inform parents/caregivers of your concerns and the next steps to be taken, unless doing so may put the child or yourself at risk. When external authorities need to be contacted, the relevant details should be ready to hand, and you should contact Child Social Services first unless the issue is more immediate, and the child needs medical attention or support from the police. Make sure the details as shown in Figure 9.2 are readily accessible.

---

2 See www.cpdt.org.uk/tab02/2_4_1_0.htm.

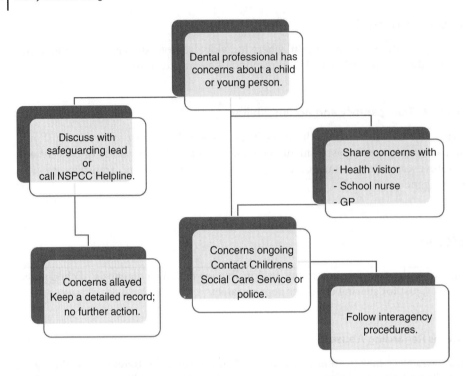

Figure 9.1 Procedures for responding to concern about child's well-being. *Source:* Figure reproduced with permission from Harris J, Sidebotham P, Welbury R et al. Child protection and the dental team: an introduction to safeguarding children in dental practice.COPDEND: Sheffield, 2006 (updated 2013). www.cpdt.org.uk, http://www.bda.org/childprotection.

CONTACT	TELEPHONE	PERSON TO CONTACT
PRACTICE SAFEGUARDING LEAD		
POLICE SWITCHBOARD	101	
CHILDRENS SERVICES NSPCC	National Helpline 0808 800500	
LOCAL SAFE GUARDING BOARD		

Figure 9.2 Emergency contact information.

Modern Slavery Act of 2015

Modern slavery is a serious and growing crime in the United Kingdom. Its victims experience one or more of the following: servitude, forced or compulsory labour, human trafficking.

A person is trafficked if she or he is brought to (or moved around) a country by others who threaten, frighten, hurt, and force them to do work or other things they don't want to do.

The Modern Slavery Act of 2015 introduced new measures and an enforcement agency to identify gangmasters and help their victims, ensuring they receive the appropriate support.

From 31 July 2015, potential victims of slavery, servitude, and forced or compulsory labour in England and Wales recognised with favourable, reasonable grounds decision may also have access to support previously only offered to potential victims of human trafficking.

Individuals who are recognised as a being a victim of modern slavery will be offered access to specialist services for at least 45 days while their case is considered, which may include:

- Access to relevant legal advice
- Accommodation
- Protection
- Independent emotional and practical help

Support in England and Wales is currently delivered by the Salvation Army and several subcontractors. The Salvation Army will assess each potential victim to determine what assistance is most appropriate; it aims to make a primary assessment of whether an individual is or may be a potential victim of modern slavery; there are 20 general indicators. These indicators are not a definitive list, and other indicators may raise concerns.

A potential victim of modern slavery is a potential victim of a crime and should be referred to the police – on the victim's behalf if they give consent, or as a third-party referral if they don't give permission (provided this does not breach any obligation of confidence under the common law).[3]

Mental Capacity Act of 2005

When the Care Quality Commission (CQC) published the results of its first inspections in England, it becomes clear how the requirements of the Health and Social Care Act 2008 are prioritised and how the available evidence is to be interpreted. This was further clarified with the introduction of The Fundamental Standards in 2015 and the associated Key Line of Enquiry upon which the quality of dental services is measured. Issues of safety and consent are at the forefront, as outlined in the Mental Capacity Act of 2005 and consent to dental treatment – Principle 3 of the Standards for the Dental Team.

Definitions

This legislation governs decision-making for people who cannot make decisions for themselves, or who presently have the capacity and want to prepare for a time in the future when they may lack that capacity. It sets out who can make decisions on their behalf, in which situations, and how they should go about this.

Consent

Consent is agreeing to a course of action – specifically care plan or treatment regime. For permission to be legally valid, the person giving it must have the capacity to make the decision, have been given sufficient information to make the decision, and not have been under any duress or inappropriate pressure.

---

3 For more information or to report a case of modern slavery, please call the helpline 0800 0121 700 or visit the modern slavery helpline website, https://www.gov.uk/.../publications/how-to-report-modern-slavery.

The Act aims to protect patients who cannot make informed decisions. It aims to support their involvement in making decisions as far as an individual can.

Under the terms of the Mental Capacity Act of 2005, patients have a fundamental right to be provided with sufficient information, in a format they understand about their treatment options. Dental professionals should act to enable patients to make informed decisions based on a clear understanding of the probable outcomes any of the treatments they consent to, and the likely consequences of refusing treatment. Obtaining and recording appropriate consent for dental treatment is a fundamental role of the dental team.

To ensure that consistent levels of care and consent are secured, dental teams need to develop high-quality policies and procedures for providing patients with sufficient information to allow them to make fully informed decisions. At no time should any patient being placed under duress. The following five principles are set out in the Act to ensure patients can consent to treatment:

1) Every adult has the right to make health care decisions and must be deemed able to do so unless a formal assessment indicates otherwise.
2) People must be supported to decide before anyone concludes they cannot decide for themselves.
3) People have the right to make what others might regard as an unwise choice and cannot be treated as lacking capacity for that reason alone.
4) If patients show lack of mental capacity, anything done for them must be done in their best interests.
5) Anything done for, or on behalf of, people without the capacity to consent should be least restrictive of their fundamental rights and freedoms.

If a practitioner has any doubts regarding an individual patient, then it would be sensible to seek specific advice. The decision-making process should consider the views of others with interest in the person's welfare, such as a primary carer, nearest relative, named the person, attorney, or guardian. In general terms of the Act, *incapable* means incapable of one or more of the following:

- Acting on decisions
- Making decisions
- Communication decisions
- Understanding decisions
- Remembering decisions previously made

An appropriately trained dental professional must assess the patient's ability to understand the specific treatment being suggested and make an informed decision. The assessment will be based on the five principles embedded in the Mental Capacity Act of 2005. Note that an individual might be able to consent to some treatment but not to others. Dentists should consider in the first instance whether the patient can consent on their behalf to the treatment proposed. However, if the view is that the patient cannot consent, then dentists should be aware that only clinicians who have undertaken an approved training course can sign the required section 47 certificate. Dentists are advised to contact their protection organisation for advice in specific situations.

Recording patient's consent is an essential part of providing quality dental services. To support practices in maintaining active records, Care Quality Commission Support has developed a Capacity to Consent Assessment Tool. This assessment can be completed on behalf of clinicians by a trained dental nurse or care coordinator. It aims to record the patients' understanding and ability to make an informed decision.

Health and Safety Laws

Health and safety laws were introduced in 1974 following some high-profile accidents and incidents, and existing health and safety laws that were deemed not to be fit for purpose and were revoked. They were replaced with a collection of new acts that make up the Health and Safety at Work Act of 1974 (HSAWA).

The HSAWA enacted the recommendations of the Committee on Safety and Health at Work (Robens Committee), which was set up to consider the existing laws and practices relating to Health and Safety. The Robens Committee came to several conclusions:

- There was too much law.
- The laws were reactive.
- The laws were unsatisfactory and unintelligible.
- The laws overlapped.
- Jurisdiction overlapped between the bodies tasked to enforce the law.

As a result, there was a general feeling of apathy in the day-to-day implementation of safety rules. To put this right, the new Act specified the legal obligations of all concerned in a single act and appointed the Health and Safety Commission, now the Health and Safety Executive (HSE), to ensure that Health and Safety laws are observed. The HSE was given a mandate to do the following:

- Provide clear guidelines.
- Allocate responsibilities (between employers and anyone affected by the work of their business).
- Ensure that the requirements of the HSAWA are met.

HSAWA places a 'duty of care' on individuals, in addition to setting codes of conduct for employers. Under the terms of the Act, all employers are required to provide a safe and healthy environment for their employees. In brief: workplaces with five or more workers employed must:

- Provide and maintain safe equipment.
- Ensure the safe handling and storage of potentially dangerous substances (Control of Substances Hazardous to Health COSHH).
- Maintain the workplace, including means of access and egress.
- Provide a working environment for an employee that is safe and make adequate arrangements for their welfare at work.
- Provide training and supervision to ensure health and safety.
- Conduct and record a risk assessment.

Risk Assessment – Because Prevention Is Better than Cure

Forty-plus years after the recommendations of the Robens Committee were enacted in the HSAWA, the concept of risk assessment is now embedded into the UK healthcare quality management culture. The ongoing development and improvement of health care services outlined in *the Regulation 12 of the Health and Social Care Act 2008* and focuses on ways to prevent accidents or adverse incidents occurring and ensuring that when the worst happens lessons are learned, and measures to prevent reoccurrences are introduced.[4]

Official Definitions

Using the definition of an accident used by the Health and Safety Executive, an accident is 'any unplanned event that resulted in injury or ill health of people, or damage or loss to property, plant, materials or the environment or a loss of business opportunity.'[5]

Ill health, damage, and loss are not desirable incidents. Ideally, they should be avoided whenever possible. In the spirit of health and safety regulations, prevention is better than cure, and the 'go-to' technique for the prevention of undesirable events is risk assessment.

Since the introduction of the HSAWA, workplace safety has increased. Taking a proactive approach to identifying hazards (potential sources of harm or adverse health effects on a person or persons) and managing risks (avoidance of threat of damage, injury, liability, loss, or any other adverse occurrence) improves bringing benefits for the safety and well-being for staff and patients.

Risk Assessment in the Management Process

In practical terms, risk assessment is central to the management process of virtually every aspect of healthcare provision. It features in the planning, leading, monitoring, and controlling methods for quality management. All policy writing should involve an element of risk assessment, with a focus on what the policy aims to achieve, what could go wrong, and any adverse impact. Risk assessment has a part to play in:

- Team selection
- Training
- Induction
- Clinical supervision
- Communications with patients
- Financial management
- Blood and saliva management
- Computer display equipment
- Quality control

---

4 Care Quality Commission. (February 2015). Guidance for providers on meeting the regulations. https://www.cqc.org.uk/sites/default/files/20150210_guidance_for_providers_on_meeting_the_regulations_final_01.pdf.
5 Robertson, Leon S. (2015). *Injury Epidemiology*, 4th ed. Lulu Books.

In each area listed above and all others, it is important to determine:

- Who is at risk
- Any controls already in place
- The likelihood and severity of the risk

A risk assessment is a judgment about how a combination of circumstances impact on safety and wellbeing. In some cases, this judgment can only be made accurately by someone with expert knowledge. The risk assessment judgment will focus on the likelihood and severity of the harm linked to the risk.

- The likelihood of harm can be assessed as Unlikely, Possible or Likely.
- The severity of harm can be assessed as Minor, Moderate, or Major.

When the harm is assessed as being Likely and the severity Major, the activity should be suspended until control measures can be put into place to make the operation safer.

Reaping the Benefits

The benefits of risk assessments are most significant when they are conducted by people with practical hands-on experience of the area being assessed, rather than a manager or supervisor who is not engaged in the activity. Whenever possible, this activity should be covered by more than one individual, to add differing perspectives to the process. This could be an area lead, a subject expert, and an operator. Effective risk assessments are excellent investments in the welfare of patients and staff, as well as in the success of the business.

Assessment of Risk

Assessments must be conducted with advice and input from others as necessary.

Step 1: Determine Risks
Assess the extent of the risks which arise. This includes employees, visitors, contractors, and other people who may be impacted by the undertaking.

Step 2: Prevent and Control
Determine what precautions are needed to manage risks that have been identified as needing attention.

Step 3: Manage
Ensure that the control measures decided on in Step 2 are implemented by employees and are managed on an ongoing basis.

Step 4: Monitor Employee Exposure
Where the risk assessment determines it appropriate, monitor the exposure of employees to the risk factors and implement health surveillance.

Step 5: Emergencies
Prepare plans for dealing with emergencies, including accidental contact, spills, or fires. Have Material Safety Data Sheets on hand for use if needed.

Step 6: Train

Where existing qualifications/training is inadequate, arrange for training or instruction in the hazards, and use of the product. Have adequate supervision and health and safety policies and procedures.

Employers are required to provide a safe and healthy environment for their employees and must keep a record of accidents and incidents (accident book). Everyone must be encouraged to enter details of accidents as they occur possibly. Even minor incidents need to be recorded because if they are frequently happening, there may well be a need for more training or equipment review.

Hazards

Health and safety risks specific to surgeries are relatively low. Practices must identify the types of hazards that exist, the effect of these hazards, the likelihood or probability of these occurring, who may be affected, and ways of eliminating or controlling the risks.

Hazards related to offices in general are usually associated with the following:

- Fire
- Work equipment and materials
- Electricity
- Visual display units
- Waste management
- Heating, lighting, ventilation
- Manual handling
- Substances
- Slips, trips, fall
- Inadequate workspace/layout
- Stacking and storage

The effects of the above range from a minor injury, for example, cuts, bruises, sprains and strains, to more severe injuries such as burns, electric shock, prolapsed discs, broken limbs, poisoning, and even death, although this is very remote.

Some accidents are not always recognised immediately. These are classed as 'slow accidents', and they arise from health-related injuries. An example of a slow accident could be the effects of smoke inhalation following a fire. The symptoms may not be apparent immediately; however, damage could be chronic and manifest several years later.

Likelihood or Probability

Judgements need to be made as to the likelihood or probability of harm occurring; this needs to be considered for each of the listed hazards. For example, you may determine that the likelihood of a child receiving injury from a square coffee table in the centre of the waiting room floor is greater than that from the same table positioned against a wall.

Fire Drills

Every member of staff should know what to do in the case of a fire at the practice; this could save lives. The fire drill should be defined and practised at practice meetings. The procedures must be displayed throughout the practice, so that every member of the team is constantly reminded of their role in evacuating the building should a fire occur.

Everyone should know where the nearest fire exit is and how to operate the fire extinguishers and understand general safety rules:

- Avoid the use of freestanding heating appliances.
- An electrician should examine electrical circuits periodically.
- Flammable substances should be stored in lockable metal cabinets.
- Control waste paper and packing materials.
- Check premises before leaving, ensuring that ignition sources are turned off.
- Frequently test the fire alarm/bell.
- Conduct periodic fire drills.
- Install and service fire protection devices
- Train staff in the correct use of fire appliances.
- Avoid placing objects close to heat sources.
- Position information signs/notices where necessary

Work Equipment and Materials

Use information signs/notices where necessary.
Position equipment and materials correctly to avoid the risk of injury.
Provide training on the safe use of work equipment and materials.
Ensure that maintenance procedures are implemented and records kept.
Ensure equipment provided is suitable for the task.

Electricity

All electrical equipment should be regularly checked and action taken to rectify shortfalls. However, the employee also must report anything that is broken or faulty so that it can be made safe. Health and safety responsibilities do not lie solely with the employer; the law states that employees have a 'duty of care' to protect themselves and others their work affects, so they must not misuse equipment or fail to report

Ensure sufficient socket outlets are provided
Avoid the use of adapters, do not overload circuits
Ensure cables are connected safely and correctly
Replace damaged cables
Carry out visual inspections of appliances, plugs and cables, keep records
Appoint an electrician to test appliances as and when required, keep records
Do not use any damaged equipment
Switch off equipment before unplugging and cleaning
Encourage the team to report defects
Extension leads must also be examined periodically
Do not move equipment unnecessarily this may cause damage to the appliance

Visual Display Units

The design of the workstation, equipment, and general environment, together with the occupational health aspects of operating visual display units (VDUs) such as computer screens must be considered.

Waste Management

Do not allow waste materials to accumulate within the office area.
Store waste in closed areas away from patient access.
Remove packaging immediately; do not allow it to collect on floors or corridors.
Ensure all office areas are domestically cleaned daily.
Clean up spillages immediately.

Heating, Lighting, and Ventilation

Ensure offices are maintained at a comfortable temperature.
Provide suitable lighting, taking into consideration the activity taking place. Consider local lighting, for example, on desks.
Ensure adequate ventilation exists, e.g. windows can be opened, or the free flow of air is present.

Manual Handling

Assess the task being carried out.
Avoid unsatisfactory movements, for example, twisting, stooping, and reaching.
Avoid excessive pushing or pulling, ensure posture is stable and balanced.
Ask for assistance from others.
Reorganise the load, make the load smaller, make it easier to grasp, ensure the load is clean, and use mechanical aids to assist with moving.
Ensure there is sufficient space to handle the load.
Remove objects that may obstruct handling.
Assess your capabilities; do you have the strength to handle the load? Never attempt to lift beyond your own limitations.
Bend knees and crouch to the load; strong leg muscles will do the work.
Keep arms lose, reducing muscle fatigue in the arms and shoulders.
Get a firm grip on the load. Grip with the roots of the fingers and palms of the hands, and do not grip by the fingertips.

Slips, Trips, and Falls

Avoid wires and power cords trailing across the floor area around legs and feet while moving about the office or at the desk.
Replace worn and torn flooring.
Do not allow paper or debris to collect in the office.
Remove handbags and briefcases from the sides of desks; place in lockers or cupboards.

Inadequate Workspace/Layout

Do not restrict access to and exit from the treatment room.
Position equipment to allow tasks to be performed safely.
Allow for easy movement of individuals within the treatment room.
Allow for easy movement when interacting with others in the treatment room.
Ensure there are sufficient floor area, height and unoccupied space to work safely.

Stacking and Storage

Objects should be stored and stacked securely, so there is no risk of falling.
Storage shelves should be strong and stable.
Avoid storing and stacking above head height to avoid reaching and stretching.

Employee Responsibilities

Accidents can and do happen in the workplace as much as anywhere. Under HSAWA, employers and employees need to work together to prevent accidents. They must produce reports outlining vulnerabilities, the likelihood of damage, estimates of the costs of recovery, and then to take all possible preventive measures. Here are three basic measures:

1) Take reasonable care of their own health and safety and any other person who might be affected by their acts or omissions at work.
2) Be compliant with the health and safety policy in force, to enable employers to meet their obligations.
3) Do not intentionally or recklessly interfere with or misuse anything provided in the interest of health, safety or welfare.

Identifying hazards and acting to prevent harm is a legal as well as a moral obligation.

10

Customer Care

Some dental professionals argue that the patient journey is a dated concept that's losing its appeal. In some cases, this may well be true. Nevertheless, it has long been clear that dental patients are looking for much, much more than good dentistry. Those practices that have recognised the importance of making their patients feel important and appreciated in these difficult financial times seem to be the practices that retain their patient base, while others with a lesser emphasis on customer care are losing theirs.

Since delighting patients need not be costly, or time-consuming in these days of high-tech communications, once a pathway for the patient journey has been established, implementing the required processes and procedures needs only the lightest touch in respect of time and resources.

Over the years, numerous people have expressed concerns about the introduction of the technology-driven dental reception desk, much in the same way as the first automatic cash dispensers were greeted when banks first introduced them. Nowadays, the disapproval that would be expressed should any of the banks withdraw that service only goes to show how changes in our lifestyles and use of technology have affected what we want from service providers.

An essential feature of good customer treatment is consistency. Excellent experiences both raise expectations and motivate patients to recommend friends. Once high expectations for excellent service are in place, just providing very good service will disappoint. Here, the consistency of automated services has the edge. Is this likely to reduce the human touch? No, it is not; instead, it will concentrate the team's attention where it is needed and streamline to routine contacts so that patients experience these as being faster and more responsive. Here is an example of how this can work.

Steps of the Patient Journey

Step 1: Patient Search

At step 1, patients either talk to friends and family or search the Internet to find an attractive dental practice. Increasingly, when they reach a website that gives them the option to ask questions and to book an appointment, then their journey begins. If at this point, the patient has the opportunity to link the dental registration to the patient's

Dental Reception and Supervisory Management, Second Edition. Glenys Bridges.
© 2019 John Wiley & Sons Ltd. Published 2019 by John Wiley & Sons Ltd.
Companion website: www.wiley.com/go/bridges/dental

personal Facebook account, they can manage their appointments on their smartphone. Some programmes allow patients to create their dental computer records, and, if they wish, to add their photograph. This, in turn, can be linked to the practice phone system so that when they phone the office, their name, picture, and records open on the receptionist's screen, allowing the receptionist to answer the phone with a personalized greeting.

Step 2: Patient Welcome

In response to the booking, the patient receives a welcoming email that provides some useful information about the practice, including directions, the availability of parking, and the range of services and products offered at the practice. This can be followed up automatically with an appointment reminder by phone, text, or email, as per the patient's request.

Step 3: Check-in

On arrival at the practice, the receptionist will have a daily list that displays patients' photos. If the patient prefers to, he or she can use the auto check-in. Patients have the option of talking to the receptionist or using an automated touch-screen system. This can speed up the check-in process, freeing up the receptionist's time to devote to the post-assessment interaction in which the patient is more likely to have questions.

Step 4: Immediate Follow-up

After the assessment or subsequent appointments, the system will send a thank you for visiting via email. This will be a chance for patients to provide feedback on their dental experiences, in a format that will meet Care Quality Commission (CQC) compliance requirements. This also allows the practice to send the patients links to information, videos, and other apps that inform and educate.

Step 5: Additional Feedback

When treatment is complete, another chance to provide feedback, with the permission of the patients, is to post a blog or testimonials on the practice website. A couple of weeks after the completion of treatment, an email that expresses the wish, 'Hope things are going well following your procedure', can also be sent. At any time, patients can opt out from the automatic email stream.

Customer Care Strategy

The retail sector has long recognised the importance of understanding the customers' 'gut responses' to their products, image, and customer service. The understanding of our patients' dental experiences, beliefs, and needs or desires, requires information drawn from a range of sources to provide insight and build customer care strategy and drive continuously improving customer care.

In any sector, good customer service is a fundamental requirement. Although a steady flow of new patients is desirable, those patients who return to you repeatedly are a testament to the quality of care they receive. Because they are satisfied, they are likely to give recommendations leading to new patients. With each satisfied customer, your business is likely to win many more customers through recommendations

How Do you Start to Create a Customer Care Strategy?

To begin with, you need to define what matters to patients. Use this information to signpost their objectives and the standard they will use to judge the quality of customer service they receive. Only when these are clearly understood will you be able to set your strategic objectives. Then a range of techniques will need to be used to measure performance towards those objectives. This could include the following surveys:

- Annual patient surveys
- End of treatment surveys
- Telephone mystery patient surveys
- Full mystery patient experience surveys

To create a worthwhile survey, begins with the end in mind.

1) *Set your main objectives.* Define the purpose of the survey and then it will be clear what questions need to be asked.
2) *Construct the analysis.* When designing your survey consider, how you will analyse the answers? 'Closed' questions (where the respondents are asked to choose from a limited number of responses) are easier to analyse than questions that are 'open' (where the respondent can reply in any way they want). Much will depend on the volume of respondents – the higher the volume, the more important it is to have an easy method of analysing the results.
3) *Capitalize on the opportunity.* Keep in mind that as well as obtaining valuable customer information, surveys are a good way to highlight aspects of your service that your customers may not be aware of.
4) *Accept warts and all.* To benefit most from a customer survey, you need to be prepared to accept criticism.

A well-designed customer satisfaction survey will enable you to identify problems so that they can be addressed; regular customer satisfaction will prevent complacency and give you early warning on where you might be losing out to your competitors' initiatives.

Having completed the survey, analyse the results. Look for specific areas where customer service needs to be improved. Ask yourself honestly if any criticism that you receive is valid and if there anything that can be done to resolve or minimize the problem.

When an area for improvement has been identified to build your action, plan to consider the following:

- Determine whether all team members are properly trained and have sufficient knowledge.
- Assess whether existing customer care measures have the desired effect on the customer experience.

- If a customer who has completed a survey has raised a specific issue, ensure that they are contacted, and their complaint discussed- don't lose an opportunity to resolve a problem and keep a customer.
- Based on the survey results, make changes and then remeasure by issuing further surveys.

The design of your patient surveys will be continuously evolving. It is essential that the whole team plays a role in meeting patients' needs and expectations. Information gathered from patient surveys will provide an excellent management tools for balancing the needs of patients with those of the dental treatment providers.

Self-Assessment for Consistently Great Customer Service

You may consider that you have excellent customer care skills and that your every customer interaction is professional, sensitive, and patient-focused. You may be right about this; however, it's more likely that from time to time, human frailty creeps in when you are tired or under pressure. This section offers you a quick self-assessment test so that you can grade your customer care standards. If you are brave enough, it would be a good idea to complete this assessment in a quality circle or peer group and discuss the scores your colleagues award you for each category.

To assess your customer service standards, award yourself a score between 1 and 10 (10 = perfect) for the following 10 questions:

1) Do you plan and prepare for your patient interactions before the start of the working day by looking at the appointment book and preempting any possible needs or challenges your patients to bring you?
2) Do you disengage from your nonwork problems and concerns? Remember that your patients will not accept mediocre service because you have a lot on your mind.
3) Do you pay attention to your appearance? In the face-to-face customer service situation, you should make a professional impression by maintaining your grooming, wardrobe, and hygiene.
4) Are you up–to-date on the treatments and dental issues that patients will ask you about?
5) Do you have a working knowledge of practice policies and procedures? Brush up on any new policies when you have free time. The more you know about your job, the better care and service you can provide.
6) Do you listen to patients' concerns in their entirety? Even if you hear the same concerns or grumbles each day, you should know how to address the issue. Most people feel better about worries or concerns if they can adequately express them fully before getting a solution.
7) Can you forgive overly angry customers, and forget about their remarks? The customer is not mad at you personally, so do not take it to heart when a customer is rude to you.
8) Can you let customers know if they are crossing the line from nerves or anger at the situation, and have started to attack you? It is a job to listen to customer's complaints; it is not your job to be verbally abused.
9) Do you try to offer patients multiple options? Customers like to feel like they have choices, so phrase questions or offers in several different ways.
10) Do you thank your customer at the end of each interaction? The customers chose to come to your practice and spend their money there, so let them know they are appreciated.

When you have scored yourself for each question, add the scores together to calculate a score out of 100 for your customer care standard.

If you want to use this task as a self-development tool, go back to the questions with the lowest scores and consider ways to raise those scores. Do not forget to revisit the questions for which you scored highest to see how those strengths can strengthen your weaker areas.

Patients judge the customer aspects of their care in highly individual and emotional terms. When practices set customer care standards in policy and procedure and equip their team to meet and evaluate them, customer treatment becomes a dynamic and rewarding part of the working life of dental professionals.

Making Patients Feel Valued

In this economic climate, most people regularly make tough spending decisions. In some cases, they must deny themselves one necessity in favour of another. Although it's true that some top-end practices seem to be relatively unaffected by a financial recession, many saw a dramatic fall in income from elective, cosmetic procedures in the great recession of 2007 to the early 2010s. During this time, it was reasonable to ask, 'How in the United Kingdom, where 50% of the population were not regular dental patients during the previous favourable economic climate, can we attract patients into best-fit options to maintain their oral health during the current financial climate?'

Although the economy significantly recovered in the later 2010s, practices are still advised to look at offering a well-structured maintenance plan that offers patients the ability to spread the cost of their care over the year and perhaps save money in the long run. A well-priced plan will allow a patient with a good standard of home treatment to save money on two oral health checks and scale and polishing by paying a monthly direct debit to the practice plan. Although this will involve the practice in a monthly administration charge, this will be more than balanced out by the regular income and potentially the sales of home treatment products on each visit.

Plan promotion need not be based solely on a financial basis. There is also the opportunity to build in added value for patients through customer care benefits linked to a loyalty scheme. Alongside the clear value of spreading the cost of basic oral well-being maintenance, plan patients can be assured that additional measures are in place to ensure that their needs are fully recognised and understood in return for their loyalty to the practice, by opting to pay a monthly direct debit to the practice.

Presenting plans to prospective new plan patients should involve examples of how much they would have saved over the previous year on their assessments, scales (and treatment if the plan offers discounts on standard private treatment fees). This will require a one-to-one discussion with each patient. This should take place in a private most importantly a low-pressure, ethical selling environment, always making it clear that it is perfectly OK if the patient chooses not to join the plan.

Once patients are on a plan, the practice needs to go the extra mile to thank them for their loyalty. Without any doubt, every patient is entitled to the best possible standard of dental treatment. Beyond the clinical care plan, patients can be offered special discounts on home treatment products and first choice of priority appointments. This requires notes to be made about each patient's preferred appointments. Another service that can be offered to plan patients is regular updates on the latest developments in clinical and home care options.

Dental businesses need to be aware of their competitors' best offerings. These are not dental practices but the companies competing for the same disposable income those patients would spend on their dental plan. They include gyms, spas, and designer labels – companies that use their marketing to make people purchasing their brands feels 'special'. As dentistry is a highly personal business, making patients feel special and cared about is a must when asking them to commit to us and offer their undivided loyalty.

Every dental professional should be fully aware of the important building trusting relationships with their patients. Trust is a precious commodity, which is hard earned and easily lost and is the result of a range of emotional responses. This fact opens the role need for teams to include treatment coordinators to focus on creating relationships in which patients are confident in the *integrity* of their dental carers. This confidence should be further reinforced by the *fulfilment of their expectations*. When patients are assured that their best interests are paramount, they will be *empowered* to make informed decisions considering the value as well as the cost of treatment options. This is shown in the triangle of trust and is built on the following six principles.

Communication

In the beginning, it is vital to introduce the role of treatment coordinator to ensure patients understand the potential benefits treatment coordination offers them. It is important for patients to be aware of the treatment coordinator's skills and qualifications.

Patient Education

Before patients can make informed choices between their prescribed treatment options, they need to understand the value as well as the cost of treatment options. By providing patients with the opportunities to hear, see, and discuss all aspects of treatments, they will feel empowered to make the oral health decisions to secure long-term health gains. This activity should take place where their confidentiality is protected.

Protection

'Do no harm' is an established ethic of the caring professions. Under this principle, dental professionals are required to keep their education and training current, as well as to know when to consult specialists or other medical professionals when they encounter a situation that is out of their realm of familiarity. That way, they are providing the best treatment for their patients and protecting them from harm.

Respect

The preexisting relationship between the dentist and the treatment coordinator is the basis of the triangle of trust. When the patient perceives a strong bond of communication and trust between the dentist and treatment coordinator, the patient is more likely to adopt a similar approach. If the procedures followed are repetitive or overlap, this will be viewed by patients as an inability to work together, and they will lose faith in the treatment coordinator. The standard procedures, forms, and treatment plans developed for the programme are essential to ensure a seamless transfer from one dental professional to the next and show patients that each team member is a professional in their field.

Continuity

Treatment coordination is primarily but not exclusively for new patients. It is vital that records of interactions with patients are kept, preventing repetition over multiple visits/courses of treatment. The treatment coordinator should read through the treatment coordination history before each treatment coordination interaction.

At its best, treatment coordination can build confidence in the integrity of dental carers. This confidence will be reinforced when patients feel their needs have been recognised, understood, and met. When patients feel their best interests are paramount, they will feel empowered to make informed choices.

Relationship Building

I always have trouble remembering three things: faces, names, and – I cannot remember what the third thing is …

We often hear people say they have a memory like a sieve. Most of us would like to have a better memory. The good news is that there are several easy techniques we can use to improve our powers of recollection.

The ability of dental professionals to remember names, faces, facts, and figures will have a massive impact on how they are valued by their colleagues, their profession, and their patients. In many ways, we judge the worth and intelligence of others based on their ability to retain information. Some people have amazing recall of numeric information; in fact, some us can remember the phone numbers of all our friends and family but can never remember where we put our keys! Research studies have shown that chess masters who years later can remember details of previous games in detail score no higher than average in other memory tests.

Memory theorists summarise memory as being the processes of registering, storing, and retrieving information. They recognise that we use our visual, aural, and kinaesthetic senses in this process. To improve the power of memory, we need to determine which of these senses is your dominate sense so that you can make good use of your strengths while working to develop areas of weakness. In his book *Moonwalking with Einstein: The Art and Science of Remembering Everything*, Joshua Foer offers these tips for memory improvement:

- *Visualize techniques.* If your dominant sense for learning and remembering is visual, link names to visual cues. For example, if a person's name is Mary, picture her dressed as Mary Poppins. Wherever possible, blend key words you want to remember with picture or places. Memory guru Tony Buzan offers this technique in his Mind Mapping process, where you can see the links between events or ideas as they are set out in linked boxes.

- *Aural techniques.* If your dominant sense for learning and remembering is aural, you could use mnemonics to create a memorable sentence as a memory aid. For example, children learning music often use *Every Good Boy Deserves Fun* to remind them of the notes on the treble clef. This can be applied to anything from shopping to tasks to-do lists. Then by voicing the mnemonic aloud, you redouble the ability to recall the information when needed.
- *Emotional links.* When your dominant sense for learning and remembering is kinaesthetic, it is essential to recognise that we remember what has the most significant meaning to us. In many cases, the reason someone has a good recall is linked to their interest in the subject. The idea is simple; if you are interested in something, you are far more likely to remember lots of details. Our brains divide memory into two sections, working-memory and long-term memory. This is such an effective system that computers mimic it.

Some people say that our memory deteriorates with age. This may well be true, but as in all things, the use-it-or-lose-it principles apply. Added to which, plenty of younger people struggle to remember as much as they would like to.

You must begin to lose your memory, if only in bits and pieces, to realise that memory is what makes our lives. Life without memory is no life at all, just as an intelligence without the possibility of expression is not intelligence. Our mind is our coherence, our reason, our feeling, even.

Gathering Patient Feedback

Continuous improvement is now a central requirement for dental care providers. This ongoing improvement depends on teams being able to gather reliable feedback about the patient experience. Practices are increasingly using apps such as the example shown in Figure 10.1 to gather patients' ratings and reviews.

NHS practices are also required to run and submit the results of Friends and Family Surveys, so that results can be published on the NHS Options website and viewed by the general public.

The first stage of the dental care development process requires us to reflect on our abilities and know our strengths and weaknesses. How do we know how well we're doing? Feedback on our performance from patients, appraisals, and audit results is essential if we are to build a realistic picture of our abilities.

However, receiving feedback can be quite a challenge! The expression 'there's no gain without pain' is a perfect description! This section looks at why feedback on our performance is both helpful and uncomfortable and considers ways to make sure the process is as positive as possible.

Although many of us know that receiving and acting on feedback is essential to our work, it doesn't stop it from feeling like we're being threatened or criticised. Receiving feedback will often evoke memories and associated feelings of 'getting into trouble' as a child. Anxiety levels will rise as the body responds with an unhelpful 'fight-or-flight' reaction. Recognising these feelings is important, but we need to overcome them and stay in our logical 'adult' if we are going to use the feedback constructively as part of the professional development process.

Figure 10.1 Apps can be used to gather ratings and reviews.

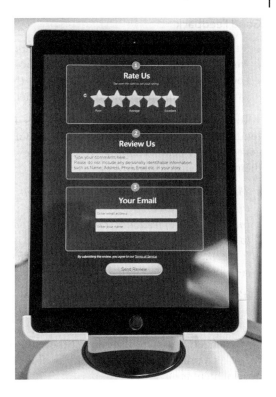

A complaining patient is unlikely to be thinking of our feelings when putting pen to paper, however, so it is vital that we can control our feelings when receiving feedback on our performance. Many patient complaints that end up at the General Dental Council (GDC) are a result of the professional being unable to make a calm and logical response to an angry letter.

Of course, the person giving feedback should also be aware of the feelings they may be evoking in the recipient. Anyone in a training or development role should be acutely aware of this. It's hard to be told we're not the perfect team member we'd hoped to be. However, when delivered constructively and with encouragement, feedback on poor performance provides the best possible development opportunities.

In our daily professional lives, we are frequently providing and receiving feedback about our interactions with colleagues and patients. Therefore, it is essential that we know how to provide constructive feedback as well as accept it. It's also important to realise that the *purpose* of feedback is to help the recipient improve their performance, not score an emotional victory. Feedback poorly delivered, or delivered with malice, can undermine confidence and becomes a disincentive for change.

So how can we learn what is good and bad feedback? Think back to a time when you have received some helpful, constructive feedback (either inside or outside work) and write down why you found it useful. Then use the same process to recall and analyse a time when you received negative feedback.

Good Feedback

- Reinforces effective behaviour, or highlights ways to improve performance.
- Aims to help the learner and not to enhance the giver.
- Focuses on a person's behaviour (which they can do something about – in other words, repeat or change) and not about their personality.

To be useful, feedback should either focus on positive, achievable changes or should reinforce behaviours you want to retain. Unfortunately, this does not match the experiences of some dental teams. Here are a few examples of the feedback they receive from their managers and employers:

- *They only ever tell me what I've done something wrong, so if my manager asks to speak to me, I fear the worst.*
- *In the absence of feedback, I'm not able to judge whether I am doing enough or doing it to the desired standard.*
- *It is demoralising when my manager only picks up on mistakes and ignores the 99% of times when things go well.*

It's a shame that such examples exist because providing good, constructive feedback is a great team builder for practice managers. The team member is likely to feel less anxious and be much happier in their work if they are supported in their professional development. They will also respect their manager, and, in turn, be more supportive of them. As a practice manager, an appraisal is probably your greatest single professional development tool.

Complaints Management

Since 2006, and the implementation of the Wilson Report, the first step for patients wishing to make a complaint about their dental care has been to seek address through the in-house complaints process at their dental practice or with the dental professional concerned.

It is hoped that through honest communication and a willingness to cooperate, win–win solutions can be agreed for most complaints without the need to involve regulatory authorities.

NHS Dental Complaints

Regulatory bodies set criteria for effective dental complaints management through programmes such as the GDC's local measures for handling the public's complaints about NHS dentists. The aim is to resolve issues at the in-house stages, rather than by the General Dental Council's fitness to practise processes. To achieve this, the policies and procedures followed by the team need to ensure that patients recognise that the team is taking their complaint seriously; and is working towards a satisfactory outcome.

If it transpires that dialogue is required between the GDC and the local NHS body that manages the contracts offered to dentists, the aim will be to ensure that the GDC deals only with fitness to practise cases while the NHS deals with other issues of performance management.

The potential benefits of this new approach include:

- A more proportionate and efficient approach in dealing with performance management issues
- Focusing GDC resources on cases where patients are at risk and a registrant's fitness to practice may be impaired
- Better use of the NHS performance management framework and using local remediation to address performance issues where fitness to practise is not impaired

Private Dental Care Complaints

The Dental Complaints service is under the umbrella of the GDC and aims to help patients address complaints about dental professionals.

They can investigate private complaints that are raised within 12 months of the treatment taking place or within 12 months of the patient becoming aware there are grounds for complaint. They will assist patients to secure the following:

- An explanation and apology for what has happened
- A full or partial refund of fees about the failed treatment
- Remedial treatment from the dental professional, if you are both in agreement
- A contribution towards corrective treatment so that the work can be completed by another dental professional at the same or an alternative practice

It's important for dental practices to recognise that there are costs involved in dealing with patients' complaints. The Dental Complaints Service alone has recovered more than one million pounds for patients. It may be that in times of health care cutbacks, patients are more likely to complain.

According to The Parliamentary and Health Service Ombudsman, the greatest number of complaints about dental services is associated with confusion about charges. This being the case, practices must ensure they have clear policies, procedures, and protocols for their team to follow.

The Ombudsman's study found that many dentists are failing to spell out the treatment patients need, to provide details on NHS and private options, or to explain the costs of treatment to patients.

The Ombudsman's findings showed that:

- The current system is confusing for both patients and dentists and can sometimes mean patients are overcharged.
- Some patients do not know whether they are entitled to an exemption from charges and fail to realise that it is their responsibility to complete the form correctly.
- Sometimes dentists fail to share treatment plans with their patients, despite an obligation to do so.

To avoid a lack of clarity that may lead to complaints, dentists need to create procedures that mean treatment options and associated costs are discussed with patients at the treatment planning stage so that patients can make informed decisions. Careful and thoughtful communication with patients is needed when outlining treatment plans to make sure the patient understands:

- The costs involved
- The likelihood of the success of the treatment
- How long a treatment will last

If the dentist considers that restoration may not succeed and last, then the patient needs to know before committing to the procedure.

This is common sense, but in a busy practice, it's easy to make assumptions about the patient's understanding of treatment. This is where the dental practitioners rely on excellent communication and teamwork skills to reduce the incidence of complaints. Prevention is the best approach to managing complaints management, by providing quality, patient-focused services that meet patients' needs and expectations.

With the focus of the dental profession firmly set upon quality and safety, dental teams are discovering three additional facts of life:

Fact 1. The more the dental profession strives to provide excellent care and service, the higher we raise our customers' expectations.

Fact 2. The more we show we are open to feedback, the more likely we are to receive criticism.

Fact 3. The process of analysing complaints is a very uncomfortable process for those concerned, which results in Interpersonal conflict.

On the face of it, these facts represent additional burdens for hardworking dental professionals, who already have the highest patient care intentions.

These points highlight the need for the development of a range of professional attitudes. This will be an ongoing process based on the quality spiral, the success of which is subject to professional and personal development and whole team professionalism.

11

Treatment Coordination

The benefits of including a care coordinator in the practice team to increase care acceptance rates are becoming increasingly apparent. This new role offers a range of benefits for patients and dental professionals as well as profitability for the dental business.

In the current health-care climate, enabling patient to make informed decisions about their care choices is a fundamental requirement. Therefore, it's a logical step for teams to include a team member with advanced communication skills and practical skills to take the care-planning process through and close the sale.

Roles and responsibilities within dental teams are regulated and permitted duties set by the General Dental Council. While it is recognised that patients benefit when dental teams cooperate, providing high-quality care must ensure that each member in the dental professional's group is providing patient care activities that are within their skills and abilities. Well-managed care coordination programmes provide excellent care development opportunities for dental professionals when they are:

- Designed to meet current regulatory requirements
- Dentist-led
- Structured
- Standardized
- Monitored and evaluated.

When care coordination involves the whole team and follows consistent clinical pathways (as shown in Figure 11.1), new and returning patients will perceive their dental visits as the pathway to better oral health, better outcomes, and better value. Care coordination provides opportunities to raise patient's dental IQs so that they can make informed decisions about their oral well-being.

The result of following these pathways will be improved efficiency and better use of resources.

Practical Considerations

Effective care coordination is a whole-team activity. Unless each team member buys in to the concept of involving, informing, and enabling patients to achieve and maintain the highest possible quality of oral well-being, any investment made by the practice to

Dental Reception and Supervisory Management, Second Edition. Glenys Bridges.
© 2019 John Wiley & Sons Ltd. Published 2019 by John Wiley & Sons Ltd.
Companion website: www.wiley.com/go/bridges/dental

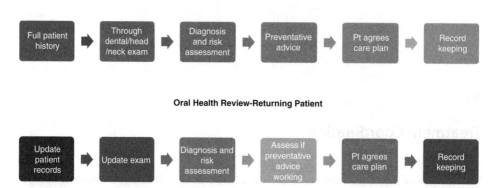

Figure 11.1 Care coordination pathways.

embed care coordination into its culture will not secure the optimum return on investment. For care coordination to meet its potential, the programme should follow these steps:

1) Set the aims objectives.
2) Define practice policy.
3) Allocate work.
4) Create procedures and working instructions.
5) Provide required material resources.
6) Train the team.

The Business Case for Care Coordination

The business case for care coordination is best made in the context of marketing and quality management. Effective care coordination is beneficial for all patient groups, and its success invariably depends on the extent to which the care coordinator knows and understands the patients' needs and expectations.

Customer Care

An essential feature of excellent customer care is consistency. Exceptional dental experiences raise patients' expectations and motivates them to recommend friends. Once high expectations for 'excellent' service is in place, providing 'very good' service will disappoint. When it comes to maintaining consistency, automated services have the edge. They always deliver to standards they are programmed to produce. Some people argue that such systems reduce the human touch, whereas others realise that if they concentrate the team's attention where it is needed and streamline routine contacts, patients consider them as being faster and more responsive. When they need information or support, their dental care coordinator is available to provide the time they need.

Raising Dental IQs – Promoting Value Rather than the Cost of Care

It is no longer acceptable for dental professionals to assume they know what's best for their patient. It is important to recognise that when a patient signs a consent form, this does not record the information used by the patient to decide to consent. Neither does it show if any undue influence was exerted to pressure the patient to reach the 'right' decision. This is why a detailed record, as would be compiled by working through a clinical pathway, is better than just a signed consent form.

The term *informed consent* is widely used, although some dento-legal bodies prefer the term 'educated consent' since it captures the fact that a patient needs to be put into a position from which they can understand the key issues, which will influence their willingness (or otherwise) to undergo a procedure.

Consent cannot be 'informed' if the patient does not understand the information provided. This could be due to the use of complex technical language or the way in which the information was presented:

- The clinician has the advantage of knowing more than the patient does, about the procedure, its risks, benefits, limitations, alternatives, and costs.
- The patient knows about their life and personal circumstances.

The care coordinator has the time and skills to ask the patient the right questions in the right way, at the right time, and will listen carefully to the patient's responses to gain an insight into whether any additional information is required.

When patients believe that they have been denied sufficient information, they often feel angry, misled, or indeed violated or assaulted. These are powerful, negative feelings that are likely to destroy any relationship of trust upon which consent is founded.

Closing Sales

When the sales interaction reaches a decision-making point, the care coordinator needs to ask the following questions:

- Do you consider that you fully understand each aspect of prescribed care?
- Are you aware of the details of care options?
- Are you aware of the benefits and possible hazards of the care plan?
- Are you aware of the costs and payment options involved?
- On this basis, are you ready to decide?

Return on Investment

There are certain costs involved in equipping a space in practice for care coordination. It is *not* ideal for care coordinators to work:

1) *In treatment rooms.* Patients will be distracted by the dental equipment surrounding them.
2) *At the front desk.* Patient confidentiality is compromised when care options are discussed in a public area.

This means that space must be set aside somewhere that the care coordinator can use visual aids to explain complicated procedures and finance options.

The practices investment will include:

- Training
- Care coordination space setup and appropriate furniture
- Necessary technology
- Staffing

This may well represent a considerable investment. Businesses will require a good return on this outlay. This return can be expected as most practices offering care coordination see substantial increases in the uptake of care plans.

Practical Considerations

In harsh economic times, excellent person-focused customer care will be well received. Using typology techniques, a skilled care coordinator will be able to profile patients and ensure the customer care approach they experience meets practice standards while taking into account the interpersonal qualities they value most.

Patient education is at the core of care coordination. Having a well-resourced care coordination space is essential. Ideally, it will contain

- Attractive lighting
- Three comfortable chairs
- Lockable cupboards
- A coffee table
- A laptop, or tablet computer loaded with the practice software
- Home care products for sale
- Literature explaining a range of procedures
- Visual aids – dentures, crowns, etc.

Working with Patients

Communication Skills

New patients should be booked with the care coordinator on their first visit for a 'getting to know you' session to cover formal introductions (see Figure 11.2). One of the aims of the care coordination interview will be to help the care coordinator to understand the patient's preferred ways of communicating. Some people are strong visual communicators and like to read or watch information, whereas others are more comfortable with the spoken word or practical activities. These preferences are influenced by character traits, personality, experiences, and education. Skilled care coordinators can pick up the cues and recognise each patient's communication needs, and then adapt their communication techniques to deliver effective communications. Before patients can make well-informed decisions, they need to be able to understand cares options prescribed for them thoroughly.

Providing Information for Decision-Making

When presenting information to patients to enable them to understand care options, it is essential to apply the central principles of learning theory. The four-stage cycle of learning includes experiencing, reflecting, thinking, and acting, in which the care coordinator interacts with the patient:

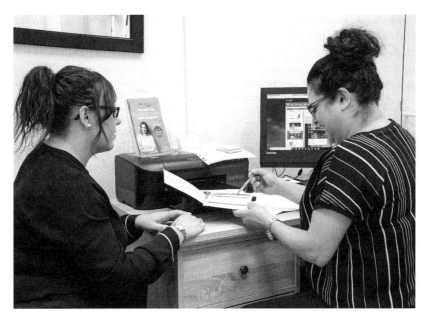

Figure 11.2 A care coordinator can provide important introductions and information to new patients.

- Information is provided to give the patients a basis for making a decision.
- Observation and reflection follow (in some cases, this means sending patients home with information).
- Information is then considered, giving rise theories.
- Options are then actively tested, possibly raising more questions.

Care Plan Scripts

Dentists are responsible for the content and quality of information provided to patients about dental procedures prescribed for patients. Each dentist will have the ways they want information presented to their patients. For this reason, each dental practice should develop pre-scripted care plans to be used for each patient.

Over the years, care coordinators learn what works best. Most find this general process to be the most effective:

- *Greeting.* Open with a greeting, such as, 'Thank you, for choosing our practice, we are happy to welcome you as a new patient. My name is ***. I am a trained/qualified care coordinator. My role is to ensure your dental experiences, at this practice fully meet your dental care needs.'
- *Engagement.* Respond to what the patients tell you about why they have selected your practice. Make it clear how the practice intends to provide good service and to listen to their point of view. It can be as simple as:
  - I'll be happy to outline how we can help you.
  - You've come to the right place.
  - Will you please tell me about your recent dental history?

- *Need development.* Ask questions so that you can understand the needs that led to the visit. This is where a full medical and dental history is taken.
- *Present solutions.* Following a full clinical assessment, explaining the details of the prescribed care and payment options.
- *Close.* Conclude the interview by repeating back what has been agreed. Review the care plan; make the appointments, the total price, and any other issues that were discussed.
- *Reinforcement.* 'We will see you again on *****, is not a very powerful end to a care coordination appointment. Try saying something more compelling, such as 'Thank you so much for being our patient. Please let us know if we can be of further help.' Or, say something that relates to the conversation, such as, 'I know you are going to be thrilled with your care.'

Preventative Home Care

The oral health educator role is central to care coordination. For patients to get the best long-term value from dental procedures, they need to have the knowledge and practical skills to enable them to control preventable oral health problems and ensure the longevity of dental outcomes.

This requirement leads to the opportunity for the sale of recommended dental products.

Appointment Planning

The lack of an effective appointments system is frequently the cause of the poor performance of care coordination systems. A poorly organised appointment book can cause chaos and result in poor relationships between all concerned.

Effective appointment planning requires a clearly defined pathway for the patient journey, from when they first decide to book an appointment at the practice, through to the successful completion of their first course of care. Procedures and processes need to be agreed and standardised, and contingency plans decided for those times when events hamper the smooth running of the process.

In both NHS and private practices, one of the primary resources requiring careful management is time, particularly the dentist's and hygienist's time. When patients are booked with more than one clinician, it is possible for the time allocations between them to become problematic.

Practical Considerations

Care quality outcomes for the involving of patients in decision making about their cares is of primary concern of care quality inspectors. There are numerous reasons why patients do not feel involved in their care decisions, ranging from a lack of intention on the part of the practice to involve them, through to difficulties the individual patient may have in understanding the information provided.

The duties of the care coordinator include a patient advocate role. By building a trusting relationship with the patient, the patient has an ally who will safeguard their best interests and they then will feel able to raise their worries and concerns with their professional friend, safe in the knowledge that they will be taken seriously, and that a full and honest explanation will be provided in terms they can understand.

Ethical Aspects of Coordinated Care

As the care coordinator role is an emerging dental team role, many teams are still defining this role and its associated responsibilities. As with any team role, the best way to identify tasks and responsibilities begins with the aims and objectives of the care coordination programme.

In many cases, the purpose of the care coordination programme can be stated as:

> To build respectful relationships with our patients. To provide the information and support to enable patients to make informed oral health choices leading to a permanent, confident, healthy smile.

Effective care coordination programme can lead to:

- Respectful carer patient relationships
- Perceptions of high standards of care
- Enlightened effective oral health choices

To run a successful care coordination programme, the care coordinator needs to be appointed, trained, and given a mandate for work activities in the format of a job description. The job description should set out:

- The overall role
- Specific tasks
- Achievement markers
- Working relationships
- Levels of discretion

Ethical Selling

Most health professionals recognise the value of ethical selling for building trusting workplace relationships. Problems occur when people define ethics too broadly and include behaviour they don't like, or behaviour that doesn't suit their own best interests, and so they accuse colleagues of beings unethical, when in fact they are basing their accusation on self-interest, opinion, or belief. This sort of view frequently arises in respect of the business–health care mix, which is relatively new to dentistry.

There can be no doubt that openness and clarity are the essences of ethical behaviour, in which clear terms are agreed with patients and only care plans directly meeting *patients'* best interests are promoted.

Informed Consent

Consent cannot be 'informed' if the patient does not understand the information provided. This could be due to the use of complex technical language, or the way in which the information was presented:

- The clinician has the advantage of knowing much more than the patient, about what the procedure involves, about its risks, benefits, limitations, about alternatives and how they compare in each of these respects, and terms of relative costs.
- The patient knows about their life and personal circumstances.

The clinician needs to ask the patient the right questions in the right way and at the right time, and needs to listen carefully to the patient's responses, to gain an insight into whether any additional information is required.

In nonemergency cases, the emphasis should be on ensuring that a patient has sufficient knowledge about the care, including:

- The purpose
- What it involves
- The likely effects and consequences
- Risks, limitations and possible side effects
- Alternatives and how they compare
- Costs

When patients believe that they have been denied sufficient information, they often feel angry, misled, or violated or assaulted. These are powerful, negative feelings that are likely to destroy any relationship of trust upon which consent is founded.

Practical Considerations

When the decision to introduce care coordination has been made, it is vital to view this activity as a whole team project. Each part of the practice has its role to play and needs to be fully involved in programme planning and development.

Training and development of practice policies and procedures are the first steps towards the consistent implementation of legal and ethical requirements. With a working understanding of regulatory and 'good practice' demands, the team can put this knowledge to practical effect within the care coordination programme.

Care Quality Standards

Patient Satisfaction Monitoring

One of the lead tasks that can be taken by care coordinators is that of patient satisfaction monitoring. A well-designed customer satisfaction survey will identify problems so that they can be addressed; regular customer satisfaction analysis will prevent complacency and give early warnings on where you might be losing out to competitors.

Patient satisfaction monitoring practices can define what matters to patients. This information can be used to signpost how patients measure dental care services and judge the quality of the customer service. This information can be gathered through the following surveys:

- Annual patient surveys
- End of care surveys
- Telephone mystery patient surveys
- Full mystery patient experience surveys

Designing Surveys

Much will depend on the number of respondents; the higher the number, the more important it is to have an easy method for analysis of the results:

- *Set the survey's objectives.* Determine what information is required and include suitable questions.
- *Pre-set analysis of the processes.* While designing consider how findings will be analysed. This will guide the choice of closed questions (where the respondents are asked to choose from a limited number of responses) or open questions (where the respondents can reply in any way they want).
- *Opportunity.* Keep in mind that as well as obtaining valuable information, customer surveys are also a good way to highlight goods and services that your patients may not be aware of.
- *Criticism.* To benefit most from a customer survey, be prepared to accept criticism.

Having completed the survey, analyse the results. Look for specific areas where customer service needs to be improved. Ask yourself honestly if any criticism that you receive is valid and if there's anything that can be done to resolve or minimise the problem.

12

Computers in Dentistry

Using Computers for Dental Administration

Like it or not, computers impact every aspect of modern life at home and in the workplace; computers make life easier for us. Computerisation in dentistry began in the larger institutions during the 1960s and gathered speed over the next 25 years. Initially, practices were offered incentives to computerise their clinical and management systems. This chapter considers security and disaster-prevention aspects of computer technology in light of recent cyberattacks and provides some simple guidelines for data protection and security.

All computers work by performing five basic operations. Competence in using computer technology begins with an understanding of these functions:

Inputting	Enter information into a computer system.
Storing	Save inputted information in a place where it can be used and retrieved.
Processing	Use computer programs to convert data into the required format.
Controlling	Direct how operations work.
Outputting	Access collated information created from the input raw data.

Data Security and Protection – NHS Practices

The quality and availability of computerized information is a significant factor in any practices ability to provide streamlined professional services to its patients. The National Data Guardian offers a range of Data Security Standards to be applied in every practice handling health and social care information, although implementation methods will vary from practice to practice. These standards set out in three obligations and 10 Standards.

Leadership Obligations and Standards

National Health Service (NHS) practices require professionals to record and audit their observation of these measures to be able to demonstrate their compliance to the regulator.

Dental Reception and Supervisory Management, Second Edition. Glenys Bridges.
© 2019 John Wiley & Sons Ltd. Published 2019 by John Wiley & Sons Ltd.
Companion website: www.wiley.com/go/bridges/dental

Leadership Obligation 1: People
Ensure staff are equipped to handle information respectfully and safely.
Data Security Standard 1:

- All staff ensure that personal confidential data are handled, stored, and transmitted securely, whether in electronic or paper form.
- Personal confidential data are shared only for lawful and appropriate purposes.

Security Standard 2:

- All staff understand their responsibilities under the National Data Guardian's Data Security Standards, including their obligation to handle information responsibly and their accountability for deliberate or avoidable breaches.

Data Security Standard 3:

- All staff complete appropriate annual data security training and pass a mandatory test.

Leadership Obligation 2: Process
Ensure the practice proactively prevents data security breaches and responds appropriately to incidents or near misses.
Data Security Standard 4:

- Personal confidential data are only accessible to staff who need it to fulfil their current role.
- Access is removed as soon as it is no longer required.
- All access to personal confidential data on IT systems is recorded and tracked.

Data Security Standard 5:

- *Processes* are reviewed at least annually to identify and improve processes that have caused breaches or near misses, or which force staff to use workarounds, which compromise data security.

Data Security Standard 6:

- Cyberattacks against services are identified and resisted.
- Security advice and action is taken immediately following a data breach or a near miss, with a report made to senior management within 12 hours of detection.

Data Security Standard 7:

- A continuity plan is in place to respond to threats to data security, including significant data breaches or near misses.
- Plan is tested once a year at a minimum, with a report to senior management.

Leadership Obligation 3: Technology
Ensure technology is secure and up-to-date.
Data Security Standard 8:

- No unsupported operating systems, software, or internet browsers are used within the IT estate.

Data Security Standard 9:

- A strategy is in place for protecting IT systems from cyberthreats, which are based on a proven cybersecurity framework such as Cyber Essentials.
- This is reviewed at least annually.

Data Security Standard 10:

- IT suppliers are held accountable via contracts for protecting the personal confidential data they process and meeting the National Data Guardian's Data Security Standards.

Staff Awareness

Practices are required to complete a staff awareness survey annually to quantify the level of preparedness for cyber incidents across the whole practice.

Audit

Arrangements for internal data security audit and external validation should be reviewed and strengthened to a level like those assuring financial integrity and accountability.

References

Report: National Data Guardian for Health and Care
  Review of Data Security, Consent and Opt-Outs
  https://assets.publishing.service.gov.uk/government/uploads/system/uploads/attachment_data/file/535024/data-security-review.PDF

General Data Protection Regulations

On 25 May 2018 new legislation came into force overwriting the Data Protection Act 1998, the new legislation being the General Data Protection Regulation (GDPR). Despite the result of the 2016 Brexit referendum, this new legislation from the European Parliament applies in the United Kingdom.

About GDPR

The GDPR follows on from the Data Protection Act (DPA) strengthening the main concepts and principles of the Act. The GDPR has considerably strengthened the rights of individuals:

- *Informed.* Data owners must be informed about the what information is held about them, how it will be used, by whom and how it is stored
- *Access.* Data owners can request access to data held about them
- *Rectification.* Data owners can require that data holders rectify inaccurately or out of date information kept about them

- *Erasure.* Data owners now have the right to be forgotten
- *Restrict processing.* Data owners can restrict processing.
- *Data portability.* Data owners can request their information to be provided to another provider
- *Object.* Data owners have the right to object to automated decision-making.
- *Automated decision-making and profiling.* Data owners can permit this.

The new regulations introduce:

- Greater emphasis on the documentation that data controllers must keep demonstrating their accountability.
- Reviewing approaches to govern and manage data protection.
- Providing individuals with more information about their data.
- Individuals rights about personal data.
- Data portability rights.
- Subject access requests.
- Obtaining consent.
- Breach notification duty.
- Privacy impact assessments (PIAs).
- The requirement for a data protection officer (DPO).

What you need to do:

1) Make sure the entire team is aware of the GDPR and its implications on their day to day work.
2) Conduct an information audit and document the personal information you hold. Record where it came from and who can access it.
3) Reinforce practice policy relating to the rights of individuals in respect of the privacy of information held about them.
4) Check practice procedures to ensure they cover individuals' rights about how data are stored and disposed of.
5) Update your systems and plan how you will handle requests within the revised timescales.
6) Review your procedures for gaining consent to hold information.
7) Review your procedures for detecting, reporting, and investigating personal data breaches.
8) Read the Information Commissioners Office (ICO) guidance about PIAs and work out how to implement these in your practice.

Emails and Messaging

Clearly defined systems for routine communication between colleagues enable individuals to work as a team. By its nature, teamwork requires the free and frequent exchange of information and ideas amongst colleagues. Irrespective of your team role, communication channels are needed to facilitate information sharing with colleagues in other areas of the practice, as quickly as if you were both in the same room.

Computers allow the team to communicate with each other discreetly. As patients arrive, a message is 'clicked' through from the reception to treatment rooms, using a function of their software of choice. For other information, the use of email and instant messaging means every member of the team can be kept up to date about events as they occur, without distracting them from their work.

Email

Electronic mail (email) is a fast and direct way to contact outside suppliers, such as labs and materials suppliers. Emails are also a convenient way to forward any referrals to specialists, leaving a clear audit trail that enables you to hold permanent records of the correspondence. Increasingly, patients prefer to be contacted by the practice by email, which is a cost-effective way to handle recalls and routine communications. It is essential to ensure that all regulations in respect to the security and protection of patient data are a fully understood band followed by each team member to avoid accidental disclosures or prosecutions.

Instant Messaging

Instant messaging can connect you to people who need or provide services. This service is provided free of charge once the software is loaded on to your computer. When the account is set up, log on to the instant messaging program using the same login name and password as for your email account.

When instant messaging is used in a dental practice, each part of the practice can be included in relevant communications. Each time you receive a new message, your computer will make a sound to attract your attention. Alternatively, you can set it to flash discreetly on the screen. As implied by the name of *instant messaging,* the message that you send arrives immediately. Emails may take a few minutes to arrive, so urgent information should be sent as an instant message.

To add other people to your messaging account, you need to know their email address. You then simply add a contact to your account and an email will be sent to them to confirm that they wish to be added to your list. When the person next signs into their messaging account, they can add you to their contacts by simply clicking to accept you as a contact.

Each time someone you have included as a contact signs into the instant messaging, you will be notified and can send them an instant response message. The advantage of instant messaging over emailing is that you do not need to keep entering the email address, or even click on reply. You can keep the message conversation open all day, or for as long as both people are signed in. Your conversation will be shown on the screen so you will have a record of what has been sent.

Once you are confident about using these communication channels, they make a positive contribution to the smooth running of the practice, making it possible for information to be shared quickly and easily.

Health and Safety Issues when Using Computers at Work

Health and safety legislation relevant to computer users is set out in an extension to health and safety law introduced on 1 January 1993. The Health and Safety (Display Screen Equipment) Regulations are in line with other health and safety regulations for electrical equipment and specifically cover workstation comfort and the long-term effect on the operator of spending long periods of time in front of a monitor.

To safeguard computer workers' well-being, employers must:

- Carry out a risk assessment and take steps to remedy any hazards identified.
- Ensure workstations meet minimum standards.
- Plan work to allow for changes in workers' activities.
- On request, arrange sight tests for significant users.
- Provide health and safety training.

To safeguard your well-being when working at a computer, you should:

- Adjust your chair so that you find the most comfortable position for your work. Your forearms should be approximately horizontal and your eyes at the same height as the top of the VDU screen.
- Make sure there is enough space underneath your desk to move your legs freely. Don't sit in the same position for extended periods. Change your posture as often as is practicable.
- Adjust your keyboard and screen to the most comfortable keying-in position.
- Make sure you have enough workspace.
- Arrange the screen so that bright lights do not reflect in the display.
- Make sure that the characters on your screen are in sharp focus.
- Keep the screen free from dirt, grime, or fingerprints, and use the brightness control on the screen to suit the lighting conditions in the room.

Index

Dental Reception and Supervisory Management, Second Edition. Glenys Bridges.
© 2019 John Wiley & Sons Ltd. Published 2019 by John Wiley & Sons Ltd.
Companion website: www.wiley.com/go/bridges/dental